Living The Slim Life
...have a plan, create the mind-set,
make it happen

by
Dr Julie Coffey

uberhealthblog.com

To purchase further copies of this book go to -
www.oodlebooks.com/living-the-slim-life/

Published by The Solopreneur Publishing Company Ltd,
9 High Farm Meadow,
WF9 1PB
www.thesolopreneur.co.uk

Medical Disclaimer
The information contained in this book is provided for education.
It is not intended as, and should not be relied upon as, medical
advice. The publisher and author is not responsible for any
specific health needs that may require medical supervision. If you
have any underlying health problems, or have any doubts about
the advice contained in this book, you should contact a qualified
medical, dietary, or other appropriate professional.
The Solopreneur Publishing Company Ltd focuses on the needs
of each individual author client. This book has been published
through their 'Solopreneur Self-Publishing (SSP)' brand that
enables authors to have complete control over their finished
book whilst utilising the expert advice and services usually
reserved for traditionally published print, in order to produce an
attractive, engaging, quality product. Please note, however, that
final editorial decisions and approval rested with the author. The
publisher takes no responsibility for the accuracy of the content.

ISBN 978-0-9930569-0-1

Printed in the U.K. by Charlesworth Press, Flanshaw Lane,
Wakefield WF2 9LP

Contents

Acknowledgements

How to get the best out of this book

Introduction

Part 1 – Out with the old, in with the new
1. Why should you lose weight?
   - What do you do when your car goes wrong?
   - The stick before the carrot
   - How have you got into this mess?
   - Rubbing some salt in
2. The problem with diets
   - Calorie restriction
   - Low fat
   - Calorie (points) counting
   - Muscle to fat ratio is key
3. Tracking your progress

Part 2 – Mind-set
4. Who do you have to BE to be slim?
5. The two parts to your mind
6. Accepting where you are now
7. Growing new habits – the key to easy change
8. You can't hit anything unless you take aim
9. Focus – how to keep it
10. How much do you know?

Part 3 – Nutrition

11. Introduction
12. Good hydration is essential to fat loss
13. Your tiny helpers – the essential nutrients
14. An introduction to carbohydrates
15. Wheat is not your friend
16. Changes to make with carbs
17. An insight into the food industry
18. Are you addicted?
19. Fat
20. Protein

Part 4 – Exercise

21. Introduction
22. Being generally more active
23. Forget about 'fat burning cardio'
24. Your 20 minute exercise plan
25. Building a bit of muscle
26. Pulling it all together

Part 5 – Your metabolism – tying things together

27. Introduction
28. How is your metabolism determined?
29. Putting the brakes on catabolic metabolism
30. How to improve your anabolic metabolism

Part 6 – Overcome comfort eating

31. Introduction
32. Comfort or emotional eating – what's the cause?
33. Dealing with comfort eating
34. Obstacles to overcome comfort eating
35. Summary

Part 7 – Keeping it going

36. 'But my life needs to get a little better before I can even start!'
37. What to do for FAST results
38. Keeping motivated
39. Summary

Food Ideas

Glossary

About Dr Julie and 'The Uber Slim Accountability Club'

Acknowledgements

My first big thank you has to go to the wonderful people who took part in my early fat loss courses. Having them to 'practice on', and having the opportunity to answer their questions enabled me to refine my message for this book. Thank you all!

The list of other writers and health experts is long, but of particular note I am grateful to the work of Andy Shaw and his Bug Free Mind Books, Dr Batmanghelidj and his work regarding water, and Udo Erasmus and his work regarding fats.

A massive thank you goes to Anne-Marie for her ongoing support and faith in me.

How To Get The Most Out Of This Book

There are only two things you need to do to get the most benefit possible from this book:

- You have to know this is going to help you (this will dawn on you as you get through the book)
- You have to read and *apply it*

At first I would suggest you relax and just read it. Don't rush to make changes or force yourself to do anything. This isn't a diet where it's all change because it's Monday tomorrow.

The whole point of this book is to correct your thinking when it comes to your health and fat loss. When you're in the process of doing that you can begin to successfully correct the mistakes you have been making, and move closer to being healthy and slim.

You won't be able to absorb everything in this book with just one read through. It's a good idea to go back through the bits you didn't get the first time around. This is particularly important in the sections about mind-set and comfort eating. Repetition is important in these sections.

You're not reading this book for enjoyment or entertainment; you're reading it to learn how to change your life. You are about to embark on a process of change. This is not just about weight loss, this is about changing your life, and it can't be approached as a race (like diets try to make it). That said, it is possible to make some big changes and see some great results in the first few weeks, but it will take months to cement these in so they become part of you and permanent. Following the lessons in this book will eventually give you certainty that you will never have a weight problem again.

A lot of people go for the seemingly short-cut: a diet. You're reading this because you know they don't work. Diets that promise things that seem too good to be true are rarely all they're cracked up to be.

What you've got in your hands is your short-cut, disguised as the long route. Because unless you change your thinking and habits you will continue to make the same mistakes over and over again, and make no progress. In two, three and five years' time, you could still be struggling with your weight.

The best way to use this book is to read it with a highlighter in your hand. Highlight all the bits that are new to you that make you think. Highlight any bit you don't agree with; you might want to ask me about them. This will concentrate your focus where it needs to be, i.e. the bits where you need to make changes or where you need to think more. It will also make it easier later when you're reviewing the book.
Write any questions or comments in the margins as

you think of them, or ideas of how you can put this into practice in your life. Engage with the book - think about what you're reading. This helps you learn. This book is yours, and by the time you've finished with it, it shouldn't be fit for someone else to read. If you've really thought about it as you've read it, it will be covered in highlights and have notes all over the margins.

By all means, read this book through quickly once, just to give yourself an overview. But don't leave it at that. The best way to read it is slowly. This gives you a chance to think as you go along. It's your thinking that will get you the results you're looking for, not speed reading.

It's also a MUST to get a notebook to write in as you go along, or you could set up a file on your computer if you prefer. As you get into the book it will be apparent why you need this.

At the end of the book you can decide whether to invest further in your health by joining Uber Slim Club. You can find more details about that here: http://uberhealthblog.com/uber-slim-club/

Uber Slim Club is hosted by Dr Julie Coffey every week and she will answer all your burning questions and keep you motivated to achieve your weight loss.

Let's get started.

Introduction

At the time of writing I have 20 years' experience as a doctor, but it's only relatively recently that I have found out how to effectively help people lose weight. Until recently I went along with the 'do more and eat less' mantra, with a bit of 'eat low fat' for good measure. No wonder people used to roll their eyes at me; this doesn't work, and they knew it.

Generally doctors have little idea how to help people with weight problems. Your doctor might even be fat themselves, and if that's the case, how can they help you? We doctors haven't been given any training about helping people to lose weight. But we are given guidelines about what advice to give people. Unfortunately these are faulty, especially when it comes to the low fat message.

So even if you follow the weight loss advice you'll receive from most doctors you're likely to fail. This might leave you thinking there's something wrong with you, when in actual fact, most doctors don't know what they're talking about when it comes to weight loss. Maybe one day we'll get taught about this at medical school, but I'm not holding my breath for that to happen.

You'll understand why the dietary advice you get from your doctor isn't going to help you as you read more of this book. Also, the penny will drop why most diets don't work either.

This book is written in seven parts, each is really important for your long term success with weight loss.

1. Out With The Old And In With The New

As a doctor I see the results of poor diet and lifestyle choices every day. I see the personal disasters it inflicts on people and their families. I see these poor choices reflected in pallid skin complexions and lank hair. I see it in their excess body fat. I see it in their breathlessness caused by just walking up a few stairs. I see people hobbling about in pain because of arthritis. On a more sinister note, I see it in serious disease and illness, which shortens both quality and length of life.

In the western world people are riddled with the 'diseases of affluence'. These include type 2 diabetes, obesity, high blood pressure, heart disease, dementia and cancer. There is a HUGE contribution to the quality (or rather, lack of it) of nutrition to all these illnesses. These types of health problems aren't so commonly seen in populations who still eat a healthy human diet. All these things become more likely as your body fat goes up.

Some people say you can be fat AND fit. This is true, and if you are fit you're a lot healthier than you would be if you weren't fit – and this is true whatever your weight. There are some extremely unhealthy slim people about; I see a lot of them too! However, if you need a bit of the stick rather than the carrot you'll get that in the first part of the book. Most people view their body fat as something that is just sat there doing nothing. It certainly is sat there, but it's not sat there doing nothing – and what it is doing isn't good for your health or lifespan, and you're going to find out why.

As a GP I get frustrated at times when people seek my help for a cure for things that should never have happened because they're preventable, or they're reversible with a little change of lifestyle. By the very fact you are reading this you are obviously interested in doing this properly and getting your health back (of course, you'll get your waist back too).

Many people I have worked with have done one diet after another. This has played havoc with their metabolism and the result was further weight gain. A screwed up metabolism also makes it harder for you to lose weight, it ages you faster, and makes you more likely to get ill by suppressing your immune system. A suppressed immune system is really bad news; it makes you more likely to get cancer. Do you really want to do this to yourself anymore?

In this first section you will discover the disastrous effects some popular diets have on you. You will find out how they can actually cause weight gain and destroy your long-term health.

This first part starts laying down a foundation to start removing the 'diet mentality'. This is a BIG mind-set problem that has physical effects, i.e. potential life-long weight problems (good news for the diet industry), and a whole host of health problems to look forward to. It needs redressing for you to be healthy and slim.

You'll also learn about tracking your progress. Probably the worst way to track this is relying on what your scales show. Your body weight alone can be really misleading and often hides real progress with fat loss. There is a much better way, and you'll learn about this in the first part.

2. Have The Mind-set For Success

The most important part of your journey towards weight loss and better health is your mind-set. I advise lots of people to lose weight during my work as a GP, as it helps the particular health problem they have. I'm often pointing out the obvious; they already 'know' this, but they're not doing it. A lot of people struggle with the motivation to even get started, let alone carry on.

Another common problem is keeping the momentum going once you start on a health plan. Lots of people start, with good intentions, but can't keep going. Often though, this is because they're doing something unsustainable and unnatural to their physiology, like a diet. At some point they slip back into old habits and any weight loss they've achieved is reversed. This is just so frustrating! But worse than this (from my point of view as a doctor) – you've harmed your health.

Having the inspiration to actually start, and then the motivation to continue long term, are major hurdles for a lot of people. Once you do some work on your mind-set these aren't problems any more. The second part of this book is going to show you how to take control of this. This sets you up for success.

Once you've got your mind-set sorted you'll be able to move forward a lot easier than you have done before. And you will be able to keep going. It's then important you know what you're doing with your nutrition.

3. Nutrition
As a species we have become so far removed from healthy human nutrition that most of us don't even know what it is.

That's a quote from a participant on my online weight loss programme. She hit the nail on the head. I know this because until recent years I considered my diet healthy. Compared to a lot of people it was very healthy. After throwing myself into learning about health I realised I was feeding my body things that were doing it harm. This was reflected in some health problems I started to have, and extra pounds that wouldn't shift.

In the third part of this book you'll learn everything you need to know about a healthy human nutrition. If you don't feed yourself the raw materials your body needs, it still needs them. It will attempt to get them by making you eat more; you'll feel hungry even though you don't need more calories. Whereas, if you give your body the nutrition it needs, you'll feel satisfied.

You will also learn about how you've been fooled into thinking some foods are healthy when, in fact, they damage your health. Many modern foods can also make you gain weight by increasing your appetite. You'll be staggered at how crafty the food and diet industry are. When you think about it, is it really in their interest that everyone gets slim? Of course not - where would their business and profits come from then?

4. Exercise

You might not be a lover of exercise. I'm not either. You don't need to be to do some, but you can enjoy the benefits.

I'm commonly given two reasons from people for not

doing any exercise.

A lot just don't like it and don't want to do it. For those of you who want the best results, and to feel great, you have to overcome this hurdle. This is where the mind-set work will be invaluable. You're also going to be really surprised just how easy it is to get started with this.

The second reason is time. Many busy people say they just haven't got the time to fit exercise in. There's good news here. With new research into exercise this one doesn't wash anymore. In part four you'll see that the most effective exercise for weight loss and health improvement can be done and dusted within twenty minutes. You'll learn how short bouts of exercise, three to four times each week, will fast track your results – both fat loss and better health.

All you need to do is keep these great changes going; you'll be able to do that because of the all-important mind-set changes you'll have made.

5. Your Metabolism
This part ties together what you'll have learned about nutrition and exercise, because what you choose to eat and do determines this. Most people think their metabolism is all about how fast they burn calories. Whilst it does have something to do with this, it's about so much more.

The quality of your metabolism reflects not only your weight, but the quality of your overall health. It's a major factor when it comes to your longevity, i.e. how long you'll live. You can't enjoy great health if you've neglected your metabolism, especially from years of dieting. When your metabolism is out of shape you're left wide open to illness and disease, which can shorten your life.

Once you repair your metabolism you will not only lose your excess body fat, but you'll also feel full of life, and perhaps even start repairing some health problems you may have. All you have to do is start working in harmony with your body, rather than against it.

6. Emotional Eating

This is such a big area for some people. In fact, if you ever eat when you're not hungry, or eat beyond feeling full (who doesn't sometimes?), you'll gain from this section.

Everything you eat starts with a decision, and being hungry might not be at the top of your list. Decisions about food are often preceded by a feeling or emotion, and these can have enormous power over your eating decisions; they're often the complete opposite to what you want.

Comfort eating results from a lack of a particular skill

that helps a person cope with their feelings. Because these feelings aren't dealt with, they're numbed with comfort food.

In this section you will be introduced to the skills you need to overcome comfort eating. These include the ability to recognise, understand and MANAGE your emotions in a way that doesn't involve eating. Learning about nutrition is really important, but if you have a problem with comfort eating that needs to be dealt with first, otherwise this new knowledge won't get you far.

7. Keeping It Going

You'll have received everything you need to successfully lose excess fat. Now it's the all-important momentum: 'keeping it going'.

This programme is not a diet that you have to stick to rigidly. It's not a diet at all. This is all about making changes that help you to become healthier, and subsequently lose weight. You don't have to be perfect. My general rule of thumb is to get it right 80% of the time and relax for the rest, if you want to. This means not getting hung up about it at all, when you eat or do unhealthy things - for example, when you go out for a meal. When you get it right most of the time your body can easily cope with some indulgences. Therefore, feeling guilty is unnecessary.

You'll learn about the areas to focus on first. Concentrating on these will fast track your fat loss results. As you go on you can incorporate more of what's in the book into your life, if you want to. You don't have to do everything in here to lose fat. But you'll know the bits you do need to concentrate on for the fastest and best results.

A lot of people who have been through this programme find they are motivated to continue because they feel so good. They feel good because they're getting healthier. Healthy bodies feel great. They also see results. You'll learn more about what you can do and what's on offer to help you even more in the final part of this book.

But in the meantime why not head over to my website and sign up for or the **free weight loss course**. You'll get weekly inspiration which will help you apply what you are about to learn in this book.

And you'll be able to email me with your questions! http://uberhealthblog.com/

Part 1 – Out With The Old, In With The New

1. Why should you lose weight?

I send out a weekly newsletter that has a link to my weekly blog. In that newsletter I asked my readers what the one big thing was that they needed help with to lose weight. I was surprised how many seemed to want to be frightened into it!

Until now, I've concentrated on getting people to focus on the benefits they'd enjoy if they lost weight. A lot of people want to improve the way they look and have more choice in the clothes they wear. They want to feel more confident or to be able to move around easier, that kind of stuff. Later in the book, you're going to be giving a lot of thought to the positive reasons why you want to change. But I do think it's sensible knowing what you're doing to your health by not taking action and losing your excess body fat.

When a person walks into my surgery with almost any long-term health problem, I see poor lifestyle choices and excess body fat as a big part of the cause. It sometimes surprises me how many people don't join the dots and see that their failing health is a direct result of unhealthy choices and being overweight.

The number of people who are overweight or obese is growing all of the time. According to UK government stats in 2012 this was the situation:

- 24.4% of men and 25.1% of women were obese
- 66.6% of men and 57.2% of women were overweight

The definitions are worked out by calculating people's body mass index (BMI); you can find more information about this in the glossary. According to these figures, people with an unhealthy body weight are becoming more and more common as time goes on.

You may already know that your weight is causing your health problems and is making you feel ill. You might already have diabetes, arthritis, high blood pressure or heart problems. You might find you're getting increasingly short of breath because of the weight you're lugging around. Maybe you sweat a lot. Body fat is a great insulator, so the more of it you carry, the more you have to sweat to maintain your correct body temperature. Think about animals that live in cold climates: seals, polar bears and whales. These creatures have to have a lot of body fat; it serves as a great insulator, keeping them alive instead of them freezing to death.

But did you know poor diet choices are the number one cause of low testosterone levels in men, and a significant cause for low mood and depression in women? Probably not. If you're like most of my patients this will come as some surprise to you, especially if you're suffering one of them and taking pills for it. It may also come as a surprise that some of the most common cancers in western countries, like breast cancer and prostate cancer, are more likely to affect you if you're overweight.

But why does all this have the increased potential to happen if you're overweight? Doesn't your fat just sit there doing nothing? No, it certainly doesn't, and when you begin to understand what it's up to, you're going to want it hanging around even less than you do now.

A wide range of illnesses can be a symptom of excess body fat. Unfortunately, the modern approach to illnesses, especially by conventional medicine, is to treat the symptoms. A lot of doctors have blinkers on when it comes to the cause of illness. There's a tendency to treat the symptoms and not cure the problem by dealing with the cause. This reflects how doctors are trained in medical school.

What Do You Do When Your Car Goes Wrong?

If you were driving along in your car and you heard a knocking sound coming from the engine, would you solve the problem by putting ear plugs in? If your oil light started flashing on the dashboard would you stick a Post-it note over it? Obviously, this is silly, because if you did that you would know the problem was still there, and it would likely get worse.

You'd take your car to a mechanic who would look under the bonnet to find the cause of the noise, and then fix it – a far better option than putting ear plugs in. By going directly to the cause and fixing it you cure the problem. Likewise with the oil light – he would check there were no leaks, fix them if there were, and top the levels up. You have dealt with the cause of the symptoms and your car can carry on in good health and run smoothly. No ear plugs or Post-it notes needed.

Health problems have a cause. That cause is often excess body fat, or at the very least, it contributes significantly. Obviously, excess body fat has its cause too, and by the end of this book you'll know how to cure that problem. If dieting sorted out the cause of excess body fat the UK (and countries like us) wouldn't have a huge weight problem. Quite clearly, dieting isn't addressing the cause.

But before we get to the cause of your excess weight some of you will want to know what your excess weight is doing to you, and I'm afraid it's not pretty.

The Stick Before The Carrot

If the 'carrot' of being healthy and looking great isn't enough to get you motivated to start changing, maybe this will give you some thought.

Far from sitting there doing nothing, your fat is quite active. One of the many things it does is produce a hormone named leptin. A hormone is a messenger. One part of the body produces a hormone and it is carried, usually via your bloodstream, to another part. This is much like an email travelling from one computer to another. Once the hormone reaches its destination it causes something to happen.

Leptin influences how hungry you are and your desire to eat. If you lose too much body fat your levels will be too low. Low levels of leptin have an effect on your brain and the result is your appetite increases. You eat more to get your fat stores back up to normal. This is a survival mechanism from the past necessary to see humans through lean times.

Humans have evolved through many years, including the ice age. This was a very lean time. It was during this time human physiology adapted to food being in short supply. You'll learn more about how this is still at work today in your body later in the book.

If you have your ideal amount of body fat your leptin levels will be low, but not too low. This is a normal, healthy state of affairs.

So what happens when you're significantly overweight

and have a lot of excess body fat? You produce a lot of leptin because you have a lot of fat; your levels are high. These high levels should turn your appetite down, but somewhere along the line that stopped happening. I'll explain why soon.

The fact is, your leptin levels are high, and this is not a normal, healthy state to be in. At high levels leptin is bad for your body – it's inflammatory. What do I mean by that? Let's look at two other things that are inflammatory: smoking and excessive alcohol intake.

Everyone knows they risk their health if they smoke. The inflammatory effect on the body makes it much more likely that the smoker will get a variety of cancers and arterial disease – leading to things like heart attacks and dementia. Excessive alcohol ages people and causes cancer and arterial disease. These are the kind of effects long term inflammation has on your body.

Anything inflammatory is essentially an irritant within your body. It causes harm to you. This harm shows itself in a variety of different ways. The effects of smoking might cause lung cancer in one person and a heart attack in another. Being overweight for years could cause high blood pressure in one person and contribute to cancer in another. If you're overweight it's like throwing a dice to see what you'll get. There is the potential for it to be many different things.

This inflammatory effect is a bit like what would happen if you left a bicycle outside in the rain instead of storing it in a shed or bringing it inside. You've left your bike in an 'inflammatory' environment. This isn't ideal for the bike, so it's going to age quicker than it would compared to if it was looked after. It becomes rusty and falls apart.

A similar thing is going on inside your body if you're significantly overweight. It's being forced to live in an inflammatory environment, so it's going to suffer the consequences. These consequences involve your body ageing quicker (like the bike going rusty) and things going wrong (like things breaking on the bike because you haven't looked after it).

A lot of people think 'It's not going to happen to me', because so many of my patients are in utter disbelief when they get seriously ill. Often, this seems to come totally out of the blue to most, yet they created the environment within their body that made it likely to happen.

As doctors we know that the more excess fat a person is carrying, the more likely they will get ill with cancer and things caused by arterial disease: high blood pressure, heart attacks, strokes, dementia (and that's not an exhaustive list).

If you're significantly overweight you're effectively

throwing the dice. What will you suffer from? Breast or prostate cancer? Heart attack? Stroke? Disabling arthritis?

Take your head out of the sand. This COULD happen to you. You're stacking the deck in favour of illness by being overweight.

When your leptin levels are raised over the long-term you suffer inflammation throughout your body as a result. This is the major reason why overweight and especially obese people are at such a higher risk of degenerative disease and illnesses like cancer and heart disease.

Carrying excess fat means you produce too much leptin. Too much leptin is the equivalent of taking an 'ageing pill' every day. This means your body is ageing quicker than it should. It might not look old on the outside but if you could take a look inside it would. Your body will be slowly breaking down and on its way to getting ill. Just like the bike rusting outside. It means you're much more likely to get an 'old age illness' early and either be incapacitated because of it or die.

I'm not being dramatic here – this is how it is. You might be thinking you knew a very overweight person who lived to a ripe old age without any significant health problems. For every one of those I'll give you a hundred who didn't. Also, this very old, overweight person may have been a very, very old person when they died if they had maintained a healthy body weight for most of their life. So don't get caught up in this sort of Muppet thinking, it's not going to help you. When other people quote this rubbish to you – smile sweetly and carry on with what you're doing.

How Have You Got Into This Mess?

What should happen when you put on too much body fat is that the increasing levels of leptin turn your appetite down. As a result you eat less and maintain a healthy body weight.

Obviously, something is happening to alter this system. There are two common reasons why:

Psychological reasons: for example, emotional eating. Many people know they eat when they're not even hungry. This might be through boredom or some kind or emotional upset. Basically, you're overriding your natural body signals when you do this. Some people do this for so long, they don't even recognise the signals their body is sending to them anymore. There's a whole section about this later in the book.

Eating unnatural foods your body has not evolved to eat. Your body is the result of millions of years of evolution. When you feed yourself what you are designed to eat, your body and its hormones will work properly. When you eat food that you're not designed to eat, your body doesn't really know how to handle it, so things go wrong and you get fat. As an example, take an avocado. This is packed with healthy fats and great for your body. Your body will love this and know what to do with it. It will not make you fat. Another example would be deep-fried chicken. This is packed with unnatural fats not found in nature. Your body will have a problem dealing with this because it's alien to what it's designed to handle. This will add to your weight problem.

You get to a point where your brain actually ignores the continually high leptin levels. To explain why this happens I'll share something I see when I take my dogs for a walk. Some dog owners shout and scream at their dogs all the time, but the dogs take little notice. The dog probably did take notice at the beginning, but because this form of communication was overused they became used to it and desensitised. They don't really hear it anymore and pretty much ignore it.

This happens to your brain when your leptin levels are too high for too long. It gets to the point where it doesn't even 'see' all the leptin floating around. It becomes completely desensitised. As a result, your brain thinks your leptin levels are really low and you're starving, and this results in your appetite increasing. Obviously, this makes things worse; ever-increasing leptin levels damage your health even more.

Rubbing Some Salt In

Your fat stores secrete many other things in addition to leptin. One thing relevant to men is an enzyme that stimulates conversion of testosterone to oestrogen. An enzyme is a very small structure that changes one thing to another. Testosterone is the 'male hormone' and is largely responsible for male characteristics.

The fatter a man is the more his testosterone changes to feminine oestrogen. This is why being overweight is a common cause of testosterone deficiency in men. It's becoming more and more common that men are complaining of the 'male menopause', and it's funny how, at the same time, men are getting fatter.

Symptoms attributed to the male menopause include low mood, lack of energy, loss of sex drive, erection problems, increased sweating, and loss of muscle mass. Less testosterone and more oestrogen in a man tips the scale in favour of man boobs too, if things weren't bad enough already.

In women, other enzymes secreted by fat cells break down oestrogen. Oestrogen is the 'female hormone'.

Women can end up with excessively low oestrogen levels that, in turn, affect serotonin action in their brains. Serotonin is a messenger in the brain, and if its action is hampered it makes depression more likely.

Treating the *symptoms* of depression and 'male menopause' (and the not the cause) is like pouring oil into your car engine without first fixing the leak. The long-term result is not going to be good.

A problem that affects men and women, of which I'm seeing more and more, is the condition 'fatty liver'. This shows up on an ultrasound scan. People have a scan on their abdomen for a variety of reasons, but a common one is because a blood test carried out to check their liver function has proved abnormal. As doctors we need to find out why.

Often, the scan comes back showing a fatty liver. Basically, the liver is full of fat; blood results come back as abnormal because the liver is under strain. It can't work properly. This can all be put right by losing weight, providing you do it in time. What could happen if you don't?

Ever heard of cirrhosis of the liver? Thought only alcoholics got that? Obesity is an increasingly common cause of cirrhosis of the liver, and it can kill you.

Another key hormone to your health and weight is insulin. Later in the book you'll learn a lot about this; I'm just going to briefly mention it here. Your hunter-gatherer ancestors had low levels of insulin. We produce insulin in response to eating carbohydrates. Hunter-gatherers ate very few carbohydrates, that's why their insulin levels were low. Low levels of insulin are both normal and healthy.

It's a completely different matter with today's carb-loaded diets. When you eat carbs your body produces insulin. The more carbs you eat, the more insulin you produce. This has consequences to your health and your weight because high levels of insulin are not normal, and therefore, not healthy.

When insulin is present in your bloodstream you lay down body fat. One of the things insulin does is cause glucose (that stems from carbohydrates) to enter your fat cells, which gets turned into fat for storage. Glucose is a simple sugar and is what all carbohydrate-based food is broken down to. When you eat food containing glucose your body has to produce insulin to deal with it. You need a mechanism to keep blood glucose levels quite low, because high glucose levels are extremely bad for you. Levels too high will kill you.

Just like the brain switching off after long-term high levels of leptin (and eventually ignoring it), the same thing happens with insulin. If you eat food that causes high levels of insulin to be poured into your bloodstream on a regular basis, eventually the cells programmed to respond to insulin stop doing so. As a result, more insulin must be produced to get the job done, which can result in high insulin levels.

At some point your body can't quite cope, and as well as your insulin levels being really high, your blood glucose levels start to go up too. Eventually, you'll become diabetic, but long before that, you will already have damaged your body with the higher-than-ideal levels of insulin in your blood. And all the time your glucose is creeping up from a normal low level to a level approaching diabetes.

Some tissues within your body can't cope with long-term high levels of insulin and glucose. Your body is the result of millions of years of evolution. It hasn't yet evolved to thrive on the modern day diet. This is why many people's health deteriorates so rapidly.

Nerve cells are extremely vulnerable to both high insulin and high glucose levels, and they suffer damage when subjected to them. This can show up as memory problems, setting the stage for Alzheimer's disease. It can also damage the nerve running from your ear to your brain, leading to hearing problems. All nerve cells are vulnerable, so the results could show up anywhere.

Other cells extremely vulnerable to high insulin and glucose levels are your endothelial cells. These are the cells lining your blood vessels. Damage to these leads to them narrowing, which has a bad effect on your circulation. Again, the results can show up anywhere; it depends where the damage is at its worst:

- Heart attack – from the narrowing and blocking of your coronary arteries (the blood vessels serving your heart)
- Strokes – when problems occur in the arteries in your neck, the ones that serve your head and brain
- Eyesight problems, including blindness – when blood vessels in your eyes are damaged
- Dementia – the tiny blood vessels within your brain narrow or even close off
- Kidney failure – the vessels to your kidneys suffer damage
- Viagra prescriptions for men – though you may seem okay everywhere else, you may not be able to get or maintain an erection because the blood vessels serving your manhood are too narrow to get enough blood there to make things work properly

This list could go on and on, but I think you get the idea. You don't have to be overweight to have trouble like this either – a rubbish diet will do, even if you remain slim. There are plenty of slim people with these health problems and diabetes. It's all down to eating the wrong things. You just increase your chances dramatically by being overweight.

Another problem with insulin is your body **cannot break fat down** while it is present. Whenever you eat something that triggers insulin you switch off fat breakdown and switch on fat lay-down. You will learn much more about insulin later.

Eating a diet that's contrary to your evolution doesn't paint a pretty picture, does it?

What this book will teach you is how to get your system running smoothly again. It's all about improving the communication and signalling between cells, by improving hormonal function. This is achieved by reducing the need for insulin and keeping leptin low. You do this by using the right type of fuel for your body. You wouldn't put diesel into your car if it ran on petrol, would you? If you did, it wouldn't work very well! The same kind of thing happens to a human body if you put the wrong fuel in.

Summing Up The Damage

The more excess body fat you carry the more you damage your health; in fact, you could be at serious risk of truly horrible illnesses.

You now know that your fat isn't sat there doing

nothing. It is, in fact, creating a hostile environment for you to live in. It's doing this by releasing hormones into your body that cause inflammation. Some of your internal organs may be suffocating under the weight of fat tissue.

I don't know if you're going to suffer the consequences of being overweight - perhaps you'll be one of the few lucky ones who suffer no ill effects at all.

But maybe you want to stack the odds in your favour from now on, and do all you can to avoid the illnesses caused by excessive body fat. You might finally be ready to tackle this once and for all, so you can be around for longer – for yourself and for those who love you.

Another way you can seriously damage your health is by going on a diet. Confused? Read on...

2. The Problem With Diets

One big problem with diets is that they tend to focus on weight loss, rather than fat loss. At the end of the day it's fat you need to reduce, and relying on your scales isn't the best way of tracking that. Despite this, it's still the thing most commonly done at your doctor's surgery.

By only measuring your weight, you don't take into

account what is actually being lost. For the sake of your health you don't want to lose weight by any of these methods:

- Dehydration
- Muscle loss
- Bone density loss

Loss of these three things will show up as weight loss on your scales. Because of your current mind-set, you might celebrate this weight loss. But how do you know if you've lost ANY fat? After all, it is fat you want to lose, isn't it? If you have a very unhealthy diet you may well lose weight from a combination of all three things, and really damage your health too. This is nothing to celebrate.

There are other things not taken into account when focusing on weight loss:

- Normal fluctuations
- Normal plateaus (your weight staying the same for a few weeks)
- Normal increases due to muscle gain

I hardly ever weigh myself, but as an experiment, I weighed myself twice a week for four weeks. I'm quite a small person, but even my weight fluctuated by four pounds in that time. If you're a bigger person your weight might fluctuate more than this.

A client of mine who successfully lost three-and-a-half stones went through plateaus lasting up to four weeks. For two to four weeks at a time she lost no weight, even though she was exercising and eating well. It took a lot of reassurance on my part that this was normal and to be expected. Fortunately for her, she wasn't only tracking her progress by her weight, and could see changes in other areas that helped her to keep going. For example, her waist measurement continued to reduce even though her weight was plateauing.

If you're someone who currently doesn't do any exercise but who then starts to, it's possible that you may put weight on. This is because you're building muscle. You may well be losing fat at the same time (which is what you want), but because muscle weighs more than fat, you could go up on the scales. Weight increase due to muscle gain is a good thing!

By continuing to be hung up on your weight you set yourself up for disappointment. Even if you're on a healthy plan like this one, chances are you're going to get upset along the way if you don't understand your weight's normal behaviour as you become healthier and lose fat. Weekly weigh-ins at weight loss clubs really are a recipe for disappointment and upset.

In fact, I'm quite happy for you to throw your scales out forever. There are much better ways of tracking real progress. You'll find out that very soon.

Calorie Restricted Diets

Human genes haven't changed in 30,000 years. This is going to cause you a big problem if you go on a low calorie diet for any length of time.

When humans were hunter-gatherers, food wasn't in constant supply. There were times when food was very scarce, and calorie intake was consequently low. What message do you imagine was sent around their bodies, via their hormones? *Famine! Food is in short supply, this is an emergency!* Humans lived in a time where death by lack of food was a real possibility. So, Mother Nature gave humans a built-in survival mechanism for when food was in short supply.

During times of calorie restriction, a human being's metabolism is hard-wired to slow down, to get through such lean periods. A few things happen:

- Fewer calories are burned – to conserve energy
- Less energy is produced – to conserve energy
- The rate of fat storage is increased – to conserve energy

These three things make it much harder to burn fat to produce energy, and much easier to lay fat down to conserve energy. This maximises your chance of survival during a lean spell. It also makes it easy to put weight on and hard to lose it.

Your genes are the same as your ancestors', 30,000 years ago. It might be the case that you are choosing to overly restrict your calories, but your body doesn't know that. Your body only perceives famine, and reacts the way it's programmed to within your genes. You can't change this.

All this causes your metabolism to slow down, and you begin to feel tired. You're less likely to do exercise and your day is going to be harder to get through. In addition, (because food is actually all around you) you're naturally going to be drawn to fast energy release foods, e.g. bread or sugary snacks. You'll learn more about these foods later, but they're the ones that don't help your waistline.

If this situation lasts for any length of time you'll need to rely on your willpower to get you through. You'll know from experience that this doesn't work. This is because it's up against two more powerful forces:
- Your in-built survival instincts – from Mother Nature
- Your habits – learned along the way, and VERY powerful (more about these soon)

But what happens if you've got great willpower and manage to keep this going for some time? Well, you're still damaging your health.

When you restrict calories your *aim* is to use the fat

on your body as energy instead. However, this doesn't happen straightaway. Even though you're not taking in enough calories to serve your energy requirements they still have to be fulfilled. Your body needs energy from somewhere to stay alive.

Initially, your body will use its glycogen stores. This is stored glucose, mainly kept in your muscles and liver. You have around seven pounds of this in storage, and if you really starved yourself you would use all of this. It's therefore possible to lose seven pounds in weight quite quickly without losing ANY fat, if you do it by starving yourself.

This is also where the weight goes from if you're ill and can't eat for a few days. Many people see this as the silver lining of being ill, but they haven't lost fat - they've just depleted their glycogen stores, which will very quickly fill back up again when they start eating.

Next, your body is going to start breaking down muscle for energy. It does this because it's easier to do this at this stage compared with breaking fat down. This is an absolute disaster, because where are most of your calories burned up – your muscles! The more muscle mass you have the more calories you burn. When you do something that reduces your muscle mass, like go on a diet, you end up with less calorie burning capability.

When you lose muscle you are losing your capacity to burn fat, pure and simple. Your muscle mass is directly proportional to your metabolic rate (which you'll learn about later). It's best to avoid anything that will make you lose any muscle mass.

It's only after you've lost some of your muscle mass that fat starts to take up the strain and is burnt as energy. Unfortunately, by this point, you've damaged your health and metabolism. Later in the book you'll learn just how important having decent muscle mass is to your overall health.

Let's remind ourselves what you do to yourself if you go on a calorie restricted diet:

- You slow your metabolism down
- You increase your fat storage capabilities
- You reduce your muscle mass

And what's worse is these effects **ARE NOT** short-lived. They don't just suddenly go back to normal when you start eating again. Your body doesn't react as quickly as a light-bulb when the switch is turned on. Your body takes a bit of time to adapt to how you treat it. These effects are long lasting, so what you've done is primed yourself for **FAST** and **SIGNIFICANT** fat gain.

This is one of the big reasons dieters pile on loads of weight, and do it really fast, after breaking their diet.

People often tell me they can't believe how fast they put the weight back on. This is an example of how adaptable your body is. The trick is to get it adapting in ways that serve your fat loss goals (and not to make you fatter than when you started).

I find it surprising when people tell me about a diet working really well for them, because they lost a lot of weight at one time. It doesn't seem to matter that they've put it all back on again. The fact is it worked because they lost two stone, so the diet must be good. They blame themselves for breaking the diet, rather than the diet itself, and putting all the weight back on. Because this is classed as success, people will do it again.

I guess this is where my definition of success is different. My definition of successful weight loss is getting down to your ideal weight and staying there long term (without suffering the misery of being on a diet).

So, many people will do the whole diet thing again and again. Either one they've done before, because it 'works', or a new one in the hope that it will work better. You can see why yo-yo dieters actually get heavier and heavier as the years go by when you understand the terrible effect it's having on their bodies.

Low Fat Diets

This is still advised by most of my colleagues, mainly because it's the advice we're given to pass on to our patients. Doctors largely trust the advice given by organisations who we assume know what they're talking about. A lot of the guidelines we doctors refer to come from NICE (National Institute for Clinic Excellence). The guidelines regarding diet for weight loss recommend reducing calories by eating a low fat diet.

Unless diet and nutrition is a particular interest of your doctor, chances are they won't have questioned this information. General Practitioners will often have an interest in a specialised area, but for the rest we rely on our training as a foundation, and the advice and guidelines given to us. I know a lot about nutrition, whereas a lot of my colleagues don't. Many of my colleagues know an awful lot more about other areas related to health than I do – in this situation I fall back on resources like NICE.

A low fat diet is just not a healthy diet for a human being. I will cover this in further detail in the nutritional section; I'm only going to give an introduction here.

First of all, have a think about what your ancestors ate. And remember that your genes are the same as theirs were 30,000 years ago. These genes evolved eating natural food. Was their diet low fat? Or was it high in fat, and high, saturated fat at that? Think about the millions of years over which humans evolved, eating a high fat diet along the way. If fat was bad for us do you think we'd have got this far? I'm talking about natural fats here, not unnatural ones, like those found in chips and pastry!

Many of the vitamins and nutrients vital to your health are found in fat. This means they're not found in naturally low fat food and they have been removed from food processed into a low fat product.

Take milk, for example. Normal full fat milk has its full complement of fat soluble vitamins – A, D, E and a very small amount of vitamin K. Moderately processed semi-skimmed milk has less of these vitamins, and full on processed skimmed milk has practically none. The more fat that's removed, the more the fat soluble vitamins disappear too. These vitamins are vital for your health:

- Vitamin A – needed for good vision and a healthy immune system.
- Vitamin D – keeps your bones and teeth healthy.
- Vitamin E – it helps keep blood flowing smoothly and reduces the chance of blood clots (which cause heart attacks and strokes).
- Vitamin K – helps you heal when you hurt yourself.

Did you know you actually need vitamins to burn energy within your body? Your body doesn't really want to consume vitamin-deficient foods, otherwise your body is more likely to store the energy you eat as fat.

Some fats are essential to ongoing good health. There are many health problems related to a deficiency in these essential fats, including obesity! Doesn't make sense, does it, but it's a fact. I'll go into this in more detail later.

If you deliberately restrict the fat in your diet you put yourself at risk, of deficiencies of both fat soluble vitamins and essential fats. Long term, both of these can make you ill and add to your weight problems.

One of the more noticeable changes I made to my own diet in my quest to get healthier was to significantly increase the amount of fat I ate. I lost weight! Years ago I was caught up in the low fat craziness; at this time I was actually at my heaviest.

The other really big problem with low fat diets is the consequential increase in sugar and refined carbs. If you take something out of your diet it has to be replaced with something else, otherwise there's hardly anything there. You'll find out later why this is incompatible to good health and your ideal weight, as well as what happens in your body when your diet contains a lot of refined carbs and sugar. In a nutshell, your appetite will increase, your insulin levels will soar, making you lay fat down. This is hardly what you're looking for.

A low fat diet goes against your genetic make-up. Your body needs fat, and it also needs the vitamins that come with the fat. And it doesn't work that well for weight loss.

Calorie (Points) Counting

Calories are pretty easy to count (though not much fun). But counting is definitely not the same as burning them.

There are several flaws with this approach:
- Vitamins and minerals are not taken into account, yet they are required to burn fat. Without them, you will struggle to lose fat.
- Essential fats are high in calories (and points) so you avoid them, yet they're needed for a healthy metabolism. Without them, you are at risk of obesity.
- Not all calories you eat are burned as energy. Some fat and protein is used to rebuild and repair parts of your body.

Calorie counting without very careful consideration to healthy nutrition is dangerous to your long-term health, and your weight.

Your Muscle To Fat Ratio Is Key

Your health and self-image has a lot to do with your muscle to fat ratio, so it's pointless talking about one without talking about the other too. Diets focus on weight loss and rarely mention muscle mass.

NEVER think weight loss. ALWAYS think fat loss.

The more muscle you have, the more energy and fat burning capacity you have. You'll feel better and have more energy.

You don't have to look full of muscles to have a good muscle mass. Muscles give definition and shape to your body. If you're a woman you'll still look very feminine with a healthy amount of muscle. You'll look toned and shapely, not like Arnold Schwarzenegger.

You'll learn how you can easily increase your muscle mass in part four of this book, even if your starting level isn't very good. Your muscles are essential for a healthy metabolism and your long term fat loss. At the very least, you need to preserve what you've got.

The thing I want you to remember is that you lose muscle by dieting. You're harming yourself when you do this and priming yourself for future weight gain.

3. Tracking Your Progress

As I've already made plain, I'm not a big fan of weighing scales. You already know that weight loss on the scales doesn't necessarily equate to fat loss, which is what you're really after.

Fat takes up to five times the space on your body compared to muscle. When done right, you lose fat and gain muscle. By relying only on the scales you're going to have some weeks where you don't lose any weight; occasionally, you may even put some on. This is normal and to be expected, but it could still feel disappointing if this is the only thing you're measuring.

The best way to track your progress is to take your measurements. At the very least, take your waist measurement. This will suffice for most men, and for women who are apple-shaped and carry most of their weight around their middle. Women who are pear-shaped (about 70% of women) and who carry their weight around their bum and thighs may find it helpful to add in hip and/or thigh measurements.

The easiest way to measure your waist is to take the measurement at your navel. The important thing is to do it in the same place every time. You want the tape measure horizontal as it goes around your body. Have a look at a You Tube video if you're not sure about this.

The other, perhaps, better way, is to do it like this:

- Find the bottom of your ribs and the top of your hips
- Breathe out naturally
- Wrap your tape measure around your waist midway between these points

The important thing is to do it in the same place each time.

You have a higher risk of health problems if your waist size is:

- More than 94cm (37 inches) if you're a man
- More than 80cm (31 ½ inches) if you're a woman

Some people do a range of measurements: upper arms, bust (or chest), waist, hips, thighs, and so on. One of my clients even measured her wrists! She had to have links taken out of her watch several times during her journey towards health.

Definitely do your waist measurement then add others if you wish. I would suggest checking your measurements every 2-4 weeks.

If you want to weigh yourself as well, that's okay, but don't do it on its own as it will hide your real progress. Do not weigh yourself more often than once every two weeks; once a month would be better. Your measurements will give you a much more accurate account of your progress.

Keep a record of this - your notebook is a good place to do that. Some people have told me they've done it on their computer; for example, on an Excel spreadsheet. Whatever works for you is fine – just make sure you keep track.

It might look something like this:

	1st Jan	1st Feb	1st March	1st April	1st May
Waist					
Chest					
Upper arms					
Hips					
Weight					
Other					

Part 2 – Mind-set
4. Who Do You Have To BE To Be Slim?

You may have managed to achieve a slim body before - perhaps several times, on this, that or the other diet. But you can't keep a slim, healthy body until you develop a slim and healthy person's mind-set. The good news is, if you learned how to walk and talk you can learn how to do this too.

When most people want to lose weight they start *doing* stuff, like changing their eating and maybe also doing some exercise. You'd do these things because you want to have something, like a slimmer and healthier body. Maybe you want to have better fitness too.

Most people fail, and you probably have too, because there's something critical missing. What I mean by 'fail' is that you either haven't lost the weight in the first place, or you've put some of the weight back on that you lost. What's missing is *who you have to BE* to be a slim and healthy person.

Your thoughts and habits HAVE to change first, otherwise you're only relying on willpower, and we all know where that gets us, don't we?

When your thoughts and mind-set change (because you've decided to change them) you become that person who consistently does the things a slim and healthy person does. As a result, you'll have what a slim and healthy person has.

When you omit the first step, i.e. who you have to be, you're doomed to failure. You can't override the person you are in your mind just by attempting to do the things that other people seem to do easily. They have a different mind-set to you; that's why it's easy for them.

The next part of this book is going to show you how you can become that slim person in your mind. You have to be that person to do what that person does to have what that person has.

5. The Two Parts Of Your Mind

One of the reasons diets fail for most people is that they do nothing to tackle the most important bit that needs to change to ensure their long term success: their mind-set.

You need to have a 'slim person's mind' before you can achieve a slim body, and keep it for as long as you're around. Until you get this bit right, you'll keep repeating the same mistakes and remain overweight or trapped in the yo-yo dieting cycle.

Your mind is quite a complicated thing, but generally speaking, there are two parts to it.

Your Conscious Mind

This is the part of your mind that you're using to read this. Basically, your conscious mind is the bit you use to be consciously aware of things in any given moment. People can't hold more than five to seven different things in their conscious mind at a particular moment in time.

At present, you'll be aware of the words you're reading - you may also be aware of any responses your reading is creating; for example, questions it's prompting you to ask. You might be totally engrossed and focused and not aware of much else right now. Or, you might be aware of several other things too, like birds singing outside. You may notice that you feel hungry, or have an awareness of being too hot or too cold.

You use your conscious mind to think. For example, when you learned to drive you had to think about it. You used your conscious mind to do this. The more you practised, the less you had to think. This was because the necessary skills were gradually being passed over to your subconscious mind.

Once you've learned a behaviour you don't tend to think about it anymore. It's then run on autopilot by your subconscious mind. This is a good thing when it comes to learning skills like driving. It's not so good when it comes to learning things that are not good for you, like unhealthy lifestyle choices.

Your subconscious mind is steered and guided by what you do with your conscious thoughts. So making some effort here will pay you back greatly later on.

Your Subconscious Mind

This part of your mind is massive compared to your conscious mind. It holds everything that you're not consciously aware of right now. Much like a warehouse would hold a huge number of things in storage, until they were needed.

Until you read this you didn't have the name of your first pet or colour of your first car in your conscious mind. But because I've directed your mind there, they've been pulled out of your subconscious mind and are now in your conscious mind.

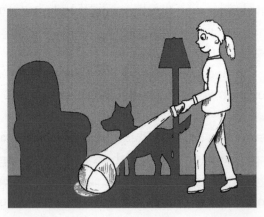

As well as storing all your memories, your subconscious stores all of your learned behaviours too. At some point, you learnt to walk and talk. You don't need to think about these anymore, you just do them automatically.

If you have children you might remember being nervous with your first baby, wondering how you were going to manage. But if you had a second, you'd have felt more confident. This is because you didn't have to learn everything from scratch. Your subconscious stored your learning from the first time around.

Let's take driving as an example. (If you don't drive, I'm sure you learned to ride a bike, so think of that.) Can you remember what it felt like when you first got behind the wheel? You might remember feeling a mixture of excitement and fear. You may have stalled the car a few times and, when you got it moving, it might have felt like you were going too fast, even though you were only doing about 15 miles an hour! You had to concentrate on every move you made; it took your full attention.

How many lessons did it take before you were able to take your test? Did you pass it first time, or did you have to retake it? How long did it take you before you felt in control and competent behind the wheel?

If you're like most people who've been driving for years

you can now do it while singing along to the radio or having a chat with the person sat next to you. You might even drive from A to B without remembering much about the journey, because you've switched off and let your subconscious learned behaviour take over.

Do you think you could have successfully learned to drive by reading one book or taking one lesson? It's pretty unlikely. It would certainly make the process a lot harder. Some people will stick with it and get there eventually, because driving is an important and necessary skill to have to them, and by persevering and learning by trial and error they'd eventually do it. But others will get frustrated and quit.

You either got there by *learning* a new behaviour (driving) and imprinting it onto your subconscious, or you didn't. When it comes to improving your health and losing fat the process is practically the same. Why is it that many people know they have to put time and effort into learning how to drive but don't perhaps realise that they have to do the same thing to learn how to be slim? I think the reason is that we've been conditioned into thinking there's a quick fix by the diet industry.

If you've seen the film 'The Matrix' you'll remember the characters could have any skill or behaviour immediately programmed into their mind. *Don't know how to do Kung Fu? No problem - a quick tap of the computer keypad and now you do; in fact, you're such an expert, you're lethal!*

If I could have learned how to drive like this I would have done, and I'm sure you would have too. So, if there's a promise of a quick fix for your weight problem most people will take it. However, by now you'll know that quick fixes don't work, and you've reached the point where you want to know why.

It's quite simple. You haven't learnt how to be slim.... yet.

I run an online weight loss course; the content of which is very similar to this book. I remember one person decided that the course wasn't for her because of the thinking effort involved. She was very honest about this - she told me she had no time to think and just needed to be told what to do. Basically, this sums up any diet. Life was very busy for her; she had priorities that were higher on her agenda than getting slim at that time.

Are you going to be like this? Or are you going to recognise that, like everything else you've successfully learned how to do, you're going to have to learn how to be slim too?

Your Reticular Activating System

You need to know how to communicate with your
subconscious mind to get it on your side, and so
it works with you towards your fat loss and health
goals. At present it's working against you, and it's
doing that because you've programmed it wrong. The
good news is that you're going to learn how to do it
correctly very soon.

There's an extremely powerful part to your
subconscious mind: your reticular activating system
(RAS). This seeks your goals like a dog follows a
scent - it keeps going until you get there. Your RAS is
working all the time to fulfil your goals. If you haven't
got what you want in life, or you keep getting what
you don't want, then you haven't programmed this
part of your mind properly.

To explain how this part or your mind works I'll use
the car as an example again. Imagine it's time to get
a new car. You decide on one you like and go and
look at it in a showroom or as a private sale. You
have a good look all round it, you sit in it, and you
take it for a test drive. You know what it looks like,
what it sounds like and what it feels like. You think to
yourself: 'That car is mine!'

Though you don't buy the car straightaway, all of a
sudden you keep seeing the same make around you -

and you especially notice the cars in the same colour than the one you've got your eye on. How can it be that all of a sudden there are loads of this particular make of car on the road? Have they suddenly just appeared, or were they there before?

They were there before; you just didn't notice them because there was no reason to. Until you decided that you wanted that particular type of car (and communicating that desire in the correct way to your RAS) your RAS wasn't programmed to bring it to your attention.

This is a really simple example of your RAS at work. You've communicated with it in a language it understands and now it's bringing these cars to your conscious attention. They were out on the road before, and although they were visible to your subconscious, it had no reason to bring them to your attention. However, now it *knows* that this is what you want, it will *bring it to your attention* whenever it can.

Your subconscious knows what you want because you've been specific about it. You've seen it, heard it, felt it. And equally as important, you've mixed some emotion in with it too. For some reason, that car is important. You may be excited because you just really want that car and you're looking forward to driving it. It might just be fulfilling a need – but you'll be clear about what that need is and you'll have thought about that too. You may have seen yourself driving to work in your new car. You know why you want the car, you know what benefit it's going to give you, and you've communicated this with your subconscious, most probably, without even being aware of doing so.

I wonder if you've gone through a similar process when you've thought about what you want, with regards your health and weight. I suspect not, because although most people use their RAS successfully in some areas of their lives they don't usually do it in all.

Further on in this section you'll learn how to program your RAS so that it helps you achieve your health goals.

6. Accepting Where You Are Now

An important part of your mind-set change is to accept where you are with your current state of health and your weight. That might sound a bit mad, because if you accept where you are now, why would you want to change?

When I explained about your RAS, using the new car as an example, I touched on how you program your subconscious mind to get what you want. In a nutshell, it involved putting your focus onto what it is that you actually want - in this case, the new car.

The thing is, you get more of what you focus on. What do you think about and say to yourself when you think about your weight? What do you feel like? Here's an extract from an email one of my blog readers sent me.

'I've been struggling with my weight since I was a teenager. I'm getting bigger and bigger as time goes on and can't seem to do anything about it. None of my favourite clothes fit me and I hate looking at myself in the mirror. I have tried every diet under the sun but none have worked for more than a few weeks. I'm fed up and totally miserable about being so overweight.'

Where does this woman have her focus at present? It's totally on the things she doesn't want.

Let's go back to the car. Imagine your current car has just about had it; it's coming to the end of its useful life or you're just plain fed up with it. It's got to the point where it's unreliable and it breaks down from time to time.

How far do you think you would get in this situation if these were your dominant thoughts about the task in hand?

'I'm fed up with this car; it keeps breaking down and making me late for work. Every couple of months I have to pay garage bills to get it fixed - it's costing me

a fortune! I don't even like the sight of this rust bucket anymore. It's just my bad luck to be stuck with a car like this.'

This might seem a bit silly, but if most of your thoughts about your car issue were along these lines, how are you going to get a new car? How are you going to move on and get something different? What it is you actually want has to be thought of first: the new car. Without doing so, you're stuck with what you've got. And then you have to communicate those thoughts with the powerful part of your mind (your RAS and subconscious) to make it happen.

So this is what happens: you decide you no longer want your current car. For the time being you accept you're still driving this car, even though you want something new. You may know immediately what kind of car you want, or you might take a while to decide. But once you decide what you want, all you have to do is make a simple plan and make it happen.

Going back to the email from my blog reader, do you think she'd accepted where she was? Of course she hadn't. And by not accepting, she was resisting. As far as her subconscious mind was concerned, she still wanted to be fat. She saw herself as fat, felt herself fat, and told herself she was fat. And then she mixed emotion with all that too: negative emotion. This way of thinking made her very unhappy. But it was the perfect way to communicate with her subconscious mind to stay overweight. Her subconscious therefore helped fulfil this goal by guiding her towards unhealthy foods, encouraging her to overeat and making her shy away from exercise. It was simply doing what it had been programmed to do, and very effectively.

By not accepting your current weight you'll instead be focusing on it. This serves as an anchor in the ground and prevents you from moving forward. If you do move forward it won't be long before you're pulled back to your starting point, i.e. overweight, or even heavier.

You don't have to like where you are now with your weight, but by accepting it you no longer focus on it. This puts you in the perfect place to focus on what you really want. What is it that you really want? Have you thought about that much?

How Do You Accept Where You Are?

You might be very unhappy with your current weight. You might also be wondering how on earth you can accept this.

An important ingredient of accepting where you are right now is knowing what you want, AND that you're going to get it. With a car that's pretty easy. Right now you might not even know what it is you want, specifically. If you do, you might doubt your ability to achieve it. The rest of this book will help you with that.

Once you know what you want AND you know you can have it you're on the road to accepting where you are now. Remember, accepting does not mean you don't want to change. Of course you want to change, you just need to take the anchor out of the ground. Non-acceptance = focus on what you don't want = getting more of what you don't want.

When you accept where you are you can feel happy. Part of this happiness is *knowing* you're no longer stuck, and that you're moving on to a slimmer and healthier body. It's about being able to look in the mirror and accept what you see, but also knowing you're moving on from it.

7. Growing New Habits – The Key To Easy Change

Human beings are, by nature, creatures of habit. You probably get up at a similar time each day, have a routine before you leave the house, and take the same route to work every day. Your socialising might involve seeing the same small number of people and going to the same places. You might go the same place every year for your holiday - perhaps even to the same hotel.

It's possible to get through most days without much conscious thought; this is because you're doing practically the same as you have done on previous days. You're on autopilot, living life by learned habits and routines. Habits are normal and can be good. It means we can learn something and then not have to consciously think about it anymore, freeing our conscious mind up to learn something new if we choose to.

These habits, however, extend to what you eat and how you use your body. If you're like most people, what you eat this week will be approximately 90% the same as what you ate last week. You buy the same things in the supermarket over and over again. You do this without much thought; this is what most people do.

This is fine if your habits and routines serve your health well, but it isn't fine if they're not. Habits can help you, e.g. taking regular exercise or hydrating yourself well on a daily basis. But habits can hurt you too, e.g. smoking or eating unhealthy foods on a regular basis.

Generally, habits make us do the same things over and over again. You may have wondered why you couldn't lose weight (and keep it off) or why no diet seems to work for you. You might feel stuck, when, in actual fact, you're not. You're simply repeating the same mistakes over and over because of your ingrained habits. It's hard to overcome these with willpower, which is why it's not normal to stick to a diet. There's nothing wrong with you, it's the diet that's the problem.

What Is A Habit?

Think about a computer or a laptop. Essentially, a functioning computer is made up of two things: the hard drive and the software. The hard drive is the physical component of the computer, but on its own it can't do anything. It needs software installed onto it. For example, most computers have Windows installed. Other examples of software are the programs that enable you to get onto the internet, use a calculator and see your photographs.

Imagine your brain as the hard drive on your computer. Like a hard drive, your brain can't do much without some software. At one time you couldn't walk or talk. You learned how to do these, so they're programmed in – the walking and talking software was successfully installed so you don't have to think about them anymore, you just do them on autopilot.

Imagine you want to speak a new language. You can't because you haven't learned it, and therefore you have no program or software in your brain to do so. It's unreasonable to expect to just pick up a new language quickly, with no effort, isn't it?

Nearly everything you do is learned behaviour from your past, including what you choose to eat and do. You have loads of deeply ingrained pieces of software, i.e. habits, and your everyday behaviour is dictated by them.

But you want different results to what you've got now. Therefore, your habits HAVE to change. Different results require different software. A computer can't do new things without the appropriate program installed, and neither can you. Well, you could give it a go and rely on willpower to get you through, but how has that worked out so far?

Going on a diet might be a habit of yours, triggered by your desire to be slimmer. If you've done repeated diets in the past, recognise this repeated behaviour as a habit; ask yourself if this habit has helped you. Is this a habit you want to continue, or change?

When you try to change your behaviour without changing the underlying habit, by installing new software, you're doomed to failure. It might work for a bit, but not long term. The smallest hiccup in your life, or just a little stress, will throw you back to your default setting: your established ingrained habit.

Unlike a computer, where you can install new

software in seconds, it takes time for you. You have to become more conscious and think about things for a while (like you did when you learned to drive), learn what to do, put what you learn into practice, and use repetition for as long as it takes. Only then will you have the new software installed and get the results you want. The old habit will be redundant.

It takes time to embed new habits. You can't rush this. It involves thinking and staying awake, rather than running on autopilot. But before you can start installing new habits you need a sense of direction.

8. You Can't Hit Anything Unless You Take Aim

Before you go any further grab a pen and write down your answer to this question: What do you want in regards to your weight and/or health? Write your answer here or in your notebook.

```
┌─────────────────────────────────────────────────┐
│ What do I want, regarding my healt and weight?   │
│                                                  │
│                                                  │
│                                                  │
│                                                  │
└─────────────────────────────────────────────────┘
```

If you don't jot at least something down you're sabotaging your success and stacking the odds against you. You're also going to miss out on learning something valuable about why you haven't succeeded so far.

If you don't do this easy thing now you'll miss out on one of the reasons you haven't got the body you want.

So write something down – anything; just put down what you want for yourself, and what you want this book to help you achieve. Write it in a way that somebody else would understand (not that you need to share this with anyone).

DON'T READ BEYOND THIS POINT WITHOUT WRITING THIS DOWN.

Before I get you to think further about exactly what you want to get out of this, imagine that you want to go on holiday, somewhere warm and sunny. You subsequently go to a travel agent and say 'I want to go somewhere warm and sunny!'

You'll likely get a blank look. The travel agent is not going to be able to help you very much with such a vague plan. 'So, where do you want to go?' the agent asks, so that he can help you book your holiday. 'There are loads of places that are warm and sunny. You could go to Spain, Florida, Greece...lots of different places.'

You decide you want to go to Greece. 'But where

exactly in Greece? There are so many places to choose from.'

You pick a particular island. Now you're getting somewhere. The travel agent begins to think you might actually know what you want.

There are still a few blanks to fill in before this holiday is going to happen, however. The travel agent needs to know exactly when you want to go, and what type of accommodation you'd like, such as a villa or hotel. As you answer his questions he collects enough information to start helping you get there, but he can only do this because you now know where it is you want to go.

But you still have a bit of work to do yourself to make this happen. How will you get to the airport? Do you need to go shopping for new holiday clothes? Do you need to organise anyone to take care of anything at home while you're gone?

Can you see the process you've gone through to achieve going on holiday? You'll have done this sort of thing numerous times. First of all, you decide what you want, and you're quite exact about that. Then you think about the steps you need to take to make it happen.

Along the way you often imagine yourself on this holiday and picture being there in your mind's eye.

You might see the clear blue sky, hear the waves breaking, and feel the warm breeze and the sand beneath your feet. You might see yourself in a nice restaurant eating lovely food and enjoying a cool glass of wine. As you do this, you'll feel good and look forward to the holiday. Any steps along the way, like the travelling, become relatively easy because you know you're going to have a great holiday when you get there.

In summary, this is what you've done:

Destination = I'm enjoying a relaxing holiday with my family on the Greek Island of Kos in an all-inclusive holiday overlooking the beach.

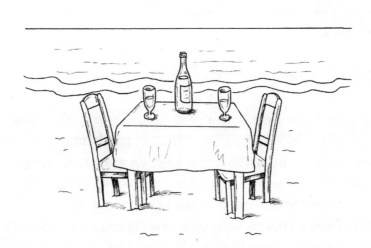

You were clear about what you wanted and can now make a plan to get there. By making a definite decision about what you want and seeing yourself there in your mind's eye you communicate with you RAS in a language it understands. This means you've engaged your subconscious and it's now working in tandem with your conscious mind. This makes getting over hurdles, i.e. the bits you might not enjoy during the process, much easier.

So, now you make your plan, which will include some of these, and probably more:

Steps:
- Book time off work
- Book the holiday with the travel agent
- Book car parking at the airport
- Organise a hire car in Kos
- Go shopping for summer clothes
- Pack

Go There Before You Get There

What I mean here is that you imagine yourself there before you actually arrive. You feel good about your upcoming holiday and look forward to it. This continues to program your subconscious. One of the results of this is that it makes potential hurdles or obstacles easier to overcome. For example, you might not enjoy the travelling or the preparation, but you do it because you know what you want and know the benefit to you.

So this is the detail you go to so that you enjoy your holiday. How much thought and detail did you go to the last time you wanted to lose weight and get healthier? I'm guessing there's a difference. Maybe this difference is part of the reason your results haven't been so good.

What's Your Goal?

Firstly, you have to know where it is you want to go, otherwise, how are you going to get there? You've got to have something to aim for, otherwise you won't hit anything. Think about walking into a travel agent and being clueless – the holiday just isn't going to happen. If you went into a car showroom and said 'I want a red car' to the salesman you wouldn't get very far. If you don't know where you're going with your weight and health, it's not going to happen either.

Secondly, once you've decided on what you want, you have to communicate it with your subconscious mind in the language it understands. Otherwise, it will keep running your existing habits, you'll feel out of control, and you'll stay exactly where you are – repeating the same mistakes over and over again.

What's your destination? Here are a few examples I've had from my patients and from people who have

taken part in my online course:
- *I don't want to be fat anymore*
- *I don't want to be a slave to food*
- *I don't want to be size 18*
- *I don't want sore knees anymore*
- *I don't want to be so unfit and out of breath*

How does your first attempt compare to these? Remember what you learned at the beginning of this section, about getting better focus? These are common ways of stating weight loss and health goals, but look at where the focus is. Your conscious mind may know what you're getting at, perhaps. But your subconscious mind is going to take you literally.

When you say to yourself something like 'I don't want to be fat anymore', what message do you think you're sending to your powerful subconscious mind? The message will be exactly what you're imagining: being fat. This is like focusing predominantly on your old car rather than deciding what exactly you want instead, i.e. a new car. You end up stuck with what you've got.

So your subconscious mind is being sent the message that you want to be fat, size 18, and have sore knees. Your subconscious will make sure it gives you what you've asked for. This is how it works. But you've seen how easy it is to get this right, and that you're doing it already when going on holiday or buying a new car.

The above examples, therefore, need a bit of work, so that your subconscious mind is engaged to help, not hinder. Here are some more examples from real people who have gone through this process:

- *To be slim*
- *I will be slim*
- *I will be in control of my eating*
- *To be fit*

Well, these are certainly a step in the right direction, but they're not very inspiring, are they? There's just no passion there - do you really mean it?

Do you think a toddler means it when deciding to walk for the first time? Of course - and so did you when you were that young. You probably didn't have the words to describe this goal, it was more seeing what you wanted and deciding you were going to have it. If you could have put words to it, it would be something like this: 'I walk!'

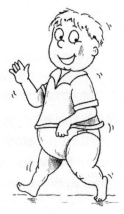

There was no mistaking what was going to happen, a powerful intention was set and you were uncompromising. There was no need to think about it or wish it could come true – it was just a done deal, and so it turned out that way.

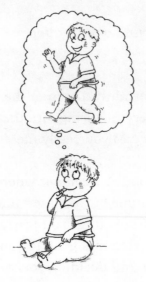

As with your goal to walk, you have to set your health and fat loss goals at a 'looking at them now' perspective. You have to 'be there' for your subconscious to get it. This is how you communicate your fat loss goals to the powerful part of your mind. Going back to the holiday – you saw yourself there in your mind's eye. With the new car – you imagined driving it or saw yourself in it before it was yours. Do the same thing with your body and your health. What do you look and feel like now you've achieved your goal?

At this stage it's not about the 'how to', so forget about that for now. When you ask a kid what they want to be when they grow up, and they say something like 'an astronaut', they're not thinking about the 'how to'. They just imagine how great being an astronaut would be.

This engages the subconscious mind. Once that's engaged you think about the 'how to', **but not before**. If you jump to the 'how to' too quickly you'll come up with all the ways you can't do it. You'll remember all the times you've failed before, you'll talk yourself out of what you're doing and quit. You need the power of your subconscious to get you where you're headed - don't stop it working for you before you even start!

Here are some reworks of what we looked at previously:
- I am slim
- I weigh x stone
- I am size 12
- I feel great
- I'm in great shape
- I'm fit
- I'm healthy
- I feel wonderful

These are short and sweet and they might be enough, depending on what it conjures up in your imagination. Taking it to the other end of the spectrum, Karen, who

took part in my course, really went to town on this
and did a great job. This was her goal:

*'I feel amazing. I have a totally amazing, fit, and
healthy body and I am my ideal weight. I have LOADS
of energy and vitality. I am flexible and lean with a
strong, strong core. My biceps and arms are strong,
lean and mean, and I have a super flat stomach with
abs to die for. My legs are lean, strong and shapely
and very, very, sexy. I look fantastic, I feel fantastic
and I absolutely love being slim, healthy and full
of energy. I feel sexy and alive and my health and
vitality shine through from every pore of my being.*

Karen's goes into some detail and when she reads it,
it makes her see her goal in her mind's eye. It helps
her 'be there now', and every time she does this she
reinforces the new program into her subconscious.
This is like having daydreams about the holiday
you're looking forward to.

Notice with all of these that they're stated in the
present. They also start with the word 'I'. When you
start any statement with 'I' it gives it more oomph;
you really mean what you're saying. You identify with
it, it's yours.

Now it's time to go back to what you wrote at the
beginning of this section. I would be very surprised
if you got yours anywhere near this yet. This bit

needs your attention and thought, otherwise it's the equivalent of asking the travel agent to book you a holiday to 'somewhere warm and sunny', or asking the car salesman for a 'red one'. You don't have to get this spot on right now, but you do have to make a start. Later on, you can tweak it and improve it if you want, but for now, improve on what you initially wrote. Start it with 'I', so it sounds like you mean it, and state it in the present tense.

Write it down here or in your notebook:

What do I want, regarding my healt and weight?

How does it make you feel when you read AND imagine your end result? It should make you feel really good. If it doesn't, you need to revisit and improve it.

Why Do You Want This?

Going back to the holiday example, if there were no reasons why you wanted a holiday, or no benefits to it, you wouldn't bother going, would you? Why would you spend all that money and go through the stress of travelling?

What would be the reasons for wanting a holiday? There may be many, and they might include some of these:

- Relaxation
- To enjoy some sunshine and warmth
- Visit family or friends
- To have fun

The thing is, when you see enough benefits and have a big enough reason why, you'll get on and do it. The benefits are clear about the holiday, that's why you do it every year. But why do you want to lose weight and/or get healthy? What's the benefit to you?

Humans are benefit-driven creatures. We don't often voluntarily do things we don't have to do unless we recognise the benefit to us. It's really important that you see the benefit of your goal you've got written down. Otherwise, you're onto a non-starter.

So why do *you* want to be slimmer?

Write your reasons down.

Here are some examples to give you an idea:

- I look great
- I feel fantastic
- I love being slim and toned
- I'm full of energy
- My body moves easily

- People tell me I look good; this feels really nice
- Knowing I'm healthy gives me great peace of mind
- My clothes fit me!

It's important that you write your own reasons down. Why is it important to be healthier and slimmer? What are all the benefits you can see towards achieving your goal? You have to know and realise the benefits of having what you want, otherwise what's the point? If there's no point there's no action towards it (at least, not for very long).

Possible Steps Towards Achieving Your Goal

So far you've got your goal written down and the reasons why you want it. Now's the time to think of possible steps to get there – the 'how to'.

Some people can't become motivated to get healthier and slimmer because the gap between where they are now and where they want to be seems too far to bridge.

What steps could you take regarding your health and weight loss goals? Start writing down a few things you could do; write anything that comes to mind, it doesn't have to be right or complete at this stage. This is work in progress.

With a holiday, because you're so used to doing

them, you might carry the steps around in your head. Equally, you could write the steps down and tick them off as you do them. It's the same thing here. At this moment in time you might not know all of the steps, but that's okay. Build it into your plan to find out what you need to know.

As you go further into this book you'll discover quite a few things that you could put into your plan. Start your plan today but expect to build on it and add to it as you go along. You might even take some things out that you've added today as your knowledge grows.

Here's an excerpt from Karen's plan to give you an idea:

- *I am learning to be healthy*
- *I am putting what I'm learning into practice*
- *I am taking small steps, one at a time, to ensure they stick*
- *Exercise is part of my daily routine; I enjoy it and look forward to it every day*
- *I have a daily yoga practice that I look forward to every day*
- *I am making healthier choices more often*
- *I am working towards cutting out all refined carbs and sugar*
- *I am reducing my caffeine intake*
- *My new healthy habits impact every area of my life in positive and healthy ways, which help to keep me going*

In this particular plan there are some pretty big changes, and they're all written in the present tense too. But just because you write things down now doesn't mean you'll do them all immediately. This is not a diet! Karen tackled one of these things at a time, and when it felt like it was part of her life and needed no further effort she started on the next one. The important thing is not to rush.

This was an early write-up. I imagine this will have been built on by now as Karen moved forward.

Thinking about, and writing down, possible steps you could take gives your subconscious something to work with. And it makes it appear possible (which of course it is). Where you are now compared to where you want to be might be a big jump. You need to give your subconscious mind some potential ways to get there, so it can mull this over and realise you can do it.

Go back to when you'd never driven a car before. There was a bit of a jump from that point to becoming the competent driver you are now. There were a lot of steps you took. Without going through these steps you wouldn't have become a good driver.

But first you had to be aware of at least some of the steps before you started. If you weren't aware of them you'd have doubted you would ever learn to drive. You started off with a few basics and added more steps as you went along, as you identified areas you needed to improve on.

By writing your potential steps down towards achieving your health goals you're doing the same thing. This massive task now appears doable, because you've given yourself a map.

Start writing your steps out, though you will be adding to them frequently. It doesn't matter how many steps you write down - in fact, the more the better.

How Good Do You Feel About Achieving This Goal?

Let's go back to the holiday example. You decided where you wanted to go, and you know why you wanted to go. The reasons why were more than enough to convince you that you wanted to go, and you knew the steps you needed to take to make your holiday happen.

Now what? Imagine being on your holiday and how good it's going to feel. Imagine the sights you might see, the sounds you may hear, maybe the sea gently coming in on the beach. A little voice in your head might say 'This feels really good'.

You have little daydreams like this quite often and they make you feel good. You know your holiday is going to happen and you feeling good about it.

Now go back to your health goal. What does this conjure up in your imagination? What does it look like? What does it feel like? What does it sound like? Jot this down. Make this personal to you, it has to make you feel good.

Here's an example from someone on my course:

'I can't tell you how good it feels to finally achieve my goal of reaching and maintaining my ideal weight. It feels so good on so many levels. I can go to any item of clothing in my wardrobe and know that it not only fits me well but looks fantastic. This feels so good and saves me so much time wondering what to wear! I absolutely love eating healthily. I look good and feel good, and when my clients and potential clients look at me they see a person they want to follow, someone they would want to emulate; it inspires trust in them as they can see that I follow what I say. It means I KNOW what I'm talking about, I don't just understand it, and this is so important to me. It's truly a blessing and possibly the best gift I ever gave myself: to put only good quality, healthy, nutritious, delicious, life-giving nutrients both into and onto my body.'

This was written at the beginning of their journey. It was written in the present tense, to communicate with the person's subconscious mind. It takes her

there in her mind's eye and engages her imagination.
By engaging your imagination and 'being there now'
you program your subconscious mind as to what you
want.

When you imagine yourself 'there', what's it like? Write
it down in your own words. What do you see, how do
you feel; what compliments will people pay you?
Writing all this down, rather than just thinking about
it, is much more powerful. If you never wrote anything
down at school you wouldn't have learned much. You
will also be reading over this a lot. You need this.

By now you'll have laid down *the* most important
part of your foundations. Without doing this, the
information in the rest of this book is not likely to
work for you. If you haven't written anything down
in your notebook, please do so before moving on.
Otherwise, you're setting yourself up for failure.

By now you should have:
- Your goal – what's your destination?
- Your 'why' – why do you want to go there? What's
  the benefit to you?
- Your steps – you need some stepping stones to get
  from where you are now, to where you want to go.
- Your 'feel good factor' – what's it like 'being there'?
  If it doesn't feel brilliant you need to start again!

What you've got written down is a BIG start. This is

not written in stone, however, and will need tweaking as you go along. At some point, though, it will just feel right.

Great work so far! Next, let's look at how to keep your focus as you move along.

9. Keeping Your Focus

Remember, you're learning new things here. To get to the point where you've *learnt* these new things, you're going to need to keep your focus on them from the beginning. If you allow your focus to slip it's inevitable that you will fall into your old ways and be back at your starting point.

People who have taken part in my course have found their notebook to be invaluable at keeping themselves on track. Some people prefer to have a physical notebook, others prefer to have a file on their computer to store this stuff. Whatever works best for you.

So far in your notebook you'll have your goal, written in a way that directs your focus to what you actually want. This is all about installing the correct software on your hard drive. It's only when you've got the correct software that you can get the results you're after.

You've also written down why you want this, i.e. the benefit to you. You'll have a written plan of how you're going to achieve this, the potential steps you may take. And you'll know how good it all feels once you've done it. This is your foundation.

The more often you look at your goal and focus on it, the more you'll be programming your mind for success. There are no hard and fast rules about how often you should do this but the absolute best way is to look at it when you get up, and when you go to bed. If this works for you, that's great, but don't beat yourself up if you don't do it this often.

The key is that when you do it, you engage your imagination, and really live your goal in your mind. Just like you would regarding the holiday or the new car. You will get little benefit by just skimming over what you've written; you have to feel it – that's how you communicate with your powerful subconscious mind. And once you've got that on your side change will come a lot easier to you.

With my own goals I'd forget to look, or not have the time to do it often. I didn't beat myself up about this (because that doesn't help), but I instead made more effort to remember. I wrote in my diary and sometimes set a reminder on my phone. I would do it most days, at least once. As it really sank in and I felt I was on my way with a particular goal I did it less often, but at least twice every week.

The more often you do it, the better, and the faster your results will happen. You're doing it right when you feel good. This means you're really engaging with your goal. You communicate with your subconscious best when emotion is involved. This is why it's so important to stop focusing on where you are right now and feeling bad about it - it just reinforces you to stay where you are.

Really get into the 'being there now' feeling. Feel good about it when you think of yourself there already – just like you would with a holiday.

There are plenty of other things for you to make a note of in your book, and every time you make an entry you're building a stronger mind-set around your health and fat loss goals.

You could put key learning points in your book. You're going to learn an awful lot as you go through the rest of this book, but you're not going to remember it all unless you interact with the book – make notes or use a highlighter pen, just like you did at school. You made notes about what you were learning. The purpose behind the note-taking was to help make it stick.

Another thing to put in your book is changes you've

made, and changes you've noticed. As you go along you'll forget some of the great changes you've made, or breakthroughs you've had. It's possible you might hit a plateau at some point and feel you aren't achieving anything. It's amazing how motivating a read through of your achievements and changes to date can be to lift you out of this state. Do your future self a massive favour and start writing things in your book now.

Here are some examples of what others have jotted down in their books:

- *It's day three of drinking more water. I've realised how dehydrated I was and have already noticed my energy levels picking up. I feel motivated to carry on with this because I can feel the benefits already.*

- *Today I had my first smoothie for breakfast. This was nice but could do with improving. It kept me full for a lot longer than I thought it would. I'll experiment with recipes.*

- *I slept really well last night, better than I can remember for years. I wonder how much this is to do with cutting down on food that isn't good for me.*

- *It was nice to eat an avocado and not feel guilty! I cannot believe I've been denying myself these things for so many years. I have also bought some nuts today and will take these to work with me tomorrow.*

- *My brother asked me if I'd turned into a health freak. Actually, I think he's jealous as I'm losing*

and he's getting fatter.
- *I didn't want chocolates at work today – weird!*

Focus on positive entries in your notebook. Remember, your subconscious mind is going to take you towards the things you focus on. However, you may want to write something negative down if it serves as a learning point. You then turn a potential negative into something positive and helpful. It would only remain a negative (and therefore unhelpful) if you didn't think it through. What do I mean by this? Here's an example to illustrate:

- *I have found it a challenge to not weigh myself every day. It almost feels like an addiction. When I'm tempted to weigh myself I remind myself that this is just an old habit that hasn't died yet. I take a few moments to focus on my goal and the bad feeling goes away. This makes me feel stronger and more confident in reaching my goal. I'm feeling more in control every day.*

This example demonstrates someone who remains aware of what's going on inside. They recognised an almost addictive feeling of wanting to get on the scales every day. They were conscious enough (i.e. not on autopilot anymore) to question this drive for daily weighing, and as a result, saw it for what it was: an old habit that was still running.

The key here is that they then switched their mind

from the old habit to their goal. In doing this, the message to their subconscious is 'No, I don't want that anymore (their addiction to weighing). I want this instead (health and fat loss goal)'.

When you do things like this you rewrite your subconscious programs and head for success. It's like loading new software onto the hard drive of your computer.

At all costs, avoid writing anything negative that you haven't turned into a positive, by giving it some thought. Here's what I mean:

- I've had a bad day today because I've eaten too much. (This focuses the mind on having a bad day by eating too much and sets you up for more of the same.)
- INSTEAD: I've had a bad day today because I've eaten too much. I think this happened because I switched off while I was eating and didn't stop until my plate was empty. Tomorrow, I'll watch out for the feeling of fullness and stop eating then. I will remain conscious while eating. (This focuses your mind on what you want to happen, rather than what has happened.)
- I have felt horrible, sluggish and fat today.
- INSTEAD: I have felt horrible, sluggish and fat today. I realise I haven't looked at my goal properly and vividly imagined my outcome for a while. I know this makes me feel good and lifts me out of

this negative state of mind. I will start doing this again every day.

Your success lies in your THINKING.

10. How Much Do You Know?

As you progress through this book you might be tempted to skim over certain parts of it. You might find yourself thinking: 'Yeah, yeah. I know this bit. Tell me something I don't know!'

Whenever you notice yourself thinking this you should sit up and pay attention, because if you do, you might learn something about yourself.

For a minute imagine there's an alien looking down at planet Earth; in particular, he's looking at western countries. He's focusing on these because they're wealthy countries yet the humans living there are often dying well before they should, and it's often related to them being overweight.

This outsider is going to come back with an answer for you to solve the growing problem of obesity.

He looked at the UK and found that, according to the public health figures of 2011, 65% of women, and 58% of men, were either overweight or obese.

He considered this problem and came up with an answer. But this answer confused him. His answer was....

- Eat well
- Exercise

You might feel insulted because the obvious has been pointed out, and it's what you know already. The alien is confused because he doesn't need to bring any cures form Mars; we have everything we need already to be slim and healthy.

One of your problems at the moment is that you know, intellectually, to 'eat well and exercise'. But because you think you know this already, you'll have a tendency to dismiss and ignore it.

But hang on a minute. You say you know this, but are you living it? If you're not living it, how can you say you know it? There's no evidence that you know it. You don't properly know how to 'eat well and exercise' until you do it.

This is an important point to remember as you read the rest of this book. When you find yourself thinking 'I know this bit', ask yourself, 'Am I applying it?' If you're not applying it, how can you say you know it? You don't. However, you can intend to apply it and make it part of your life.

You don't know it, until you're applying it.

Part 3
11. Introduction To Part 3

Warning!

Do the work outlined in Part 2 **before** diving into this part. It's highly likely that one of the biggest reasons you haven't succeeded so far is because you haven't got a slim mind-set yet. When you start putting that right you'll find making the changes detailed in this part much easier.

Without first starting to fix your ingrained habits you're highly likely to revert back to old ways. This might happen slowly without you noticing, or quickly, because it's been triggered through stress, for example. Save yourself time in the long run by putting down firm foundations before getting stuck into this part.

So, if you haven't done the work in part 2 – go back and do it before going any further.

This part is a review of what constitutes a healthy way to nourish your body. You don't have to do everything in order to be successful at losing your unwanted body fat, but the more you do the healthier you will be.

Please don't rush to try and put all this into practice

straightaway. By taking your time and doing this gradually you will massively increase your chances of success. It's best to take it one step at a time and make your changes gradually.

At the beginning of my own journey towards greater health I kept a record of all the changes I made, because I wanted to notice the impact of each one. Within the first nine months I made sixteen changes. These included things like drinking more water, taking more exercise, eating better quality snacks, reducing refined carbs. Since then I've made many more. I just keep adding changes in, in a gradual way. The ones I started at the beginning are on autopilot now, I hardly have to think about them; I certainly use no effort to make myself do them. The message here is to not rush, just keep making regular changes. Make this easy on yourself.

Most people want results as quickly as possible. With that in mind, concentrate on making changes detailed in chapters 12 - 16 first. You can improve your eating habits and food choices further as you go along, with the information in the latter half of this section.

The foundation of your health and fat loss is to hydrate yourself properly every day. Let's look at this further.

12. Good Hydration Is Essential For Fat Loss

Your body is made up of approximately 75% water, which may come as no surprise to you. Only about 10 pints of this water is within your blood circulation. But think about how much you weigh, and the fact that 75% of your weight is water. Where's the rest? The 10 pints within your blood circulation is a drop in the ocean when it comes to how much water is within your body.

There are two other reservoirs of water within your body, besides that of your blood circulation. One is within the cells that make up your body and the other is surrounding the cells (between the cells and the blood vessels; this is called lymph).

The lymph, which is mostly water, bathes the cells in liquid. It floats nutrients from the blood circulation into the cells. It works the other way around too. Waste from the cells floats over into the blood circulation so it can be taken away and removed from the body.

The cells have membranes around them, to keep them separate from each other and from the outside. There's lots of water within your cells, lots of it around the cells and a smaller amount within your circulation. Membranes can be compared to the walls of your house. There's air on either side of the walls, but the walls act as barriers. This means that the air can be different on each side, e.g. it can be kept warmer on the inside. Cell membranes are a bit like that. They keep things inside differently to what's on the outside. Water can travel across (like air can in your house), but it is controlled. This is important, because you have lots of different types of cells in your body and they need different things – one being the amount of water they need. For example, your brain cells need more water than your fat cells.

Here's something you might not know about water, in relation to your body:

As you get older your thirst mechanism gradually declines. When you were a child it worked perfectly. If your body became just a little dehydrated you felt thirsty, which would prompt you to drink. However, this will have started to change when you reached your twenties.

If you take the 25 year-old version of you and your 45 year-old version, both experiencing the same level of thirst, the 45 year-old would be significantly more dehydrated compared with the younger version. The 60 year-old version of you would be even more dehydrated. This is very clearly seen in the aged amongst us; I see it a lot in nursing homes. Residents often claim they're not thirsty, despite not having had a drink all day long. It's easy for older people to become severely dehydrated without even being aware of it.

This means, depending on your age, you might be in a permanent state of dehydration if you rely on your thirst mechanism to tell you when you're thirsty. It means that, the older you are, when you actually experience the sensation of thirst you could be significantly dehydrated. This has a lot of potential health implications, obesity being one of them. You'll see why this is so important to your fat loss efforts next.

Drinking Water Aids Weight Loss

It really doesn't get much easier than this.

I've heard lots of people say, and diets profess, that drinking water fills you up, so making sure you drink before a meal is a good way to not eat so much. This isn't entirely true, but there is something in it.

Did you know that the early sensations of thirst and hunger are very similar?

Your brain is the driving force of your fluid intake. It's made up mostly of water, about 85%, in fact. Most of the time people don't give their brain a thought, unless they've got a hangover. Then it reminds you that it's there because it hurts. It hurts because it's dehydrated.

Your brain has several energy sources. Some of the energy your brain uses is generated by water (which is, of course, calorie free) travelling across cell membranes. This is like hydroelectric energy. Your brain also uses energy by burning glucose.

Because some of your brain's energy is derived from water it will ask for more when your body is getting a bit dry. Your brain has more water in it than any other part of your body, so it's going to feel any shortage first. This is why your brain is the chief driver to your hydration.

Because no one told us that mild hunger can actually mean we're thirsty, most people eat at this point. So though your brain wanted more water for its energy it got food instead. People often eat when their body is signalling for water.

Your brain will use some of the energy from this food but the brain is a very small organ, so it's not going to use much. If you weren't genuinely hungry for calories the rest of your body doesn't need this food yet either. It's consequently destined for your fat stores.

Simply not hydrating your body enough means you could be compounding your weight problem.

Your Fat Is Not Forgotten

You might think your body fat is stuck on you doing nothing. You already know that's not true from the introduction to this book. Your fat is an active part of your body - producing hormones, for one thing. However, the fat you have now is different to the fat you had a month or two ago. Your body fat is actually recycled every few weeks. This means that, as some is laid down, other bits are broken down. It's not static on a microscopic level, although it feels like it is to you.

One of the jobs of fat tissue is to pick up excess energy from the food we eat and store it. An important role it has is keeping your blood sugar down (more about that later in the book). Your fat is always in flux – being laid down, and being broken down. Nothing in your body is static, it's always being renewed. Your aim is to tip the scales towards more 'breakdown', compared with 'lay down'.

Fat breakdown depends on water. It doesn't happen efficiently without plenty of it.

If you look at your body fat as a whole, something has to happen to it for it to shrink so you can get slimmer. It needs to be broken down into small enough units that can be transported around your system by your bloodstream, to cross over into cells and then be burned up to release energy.

An enzyme called lipase is essential to breaking down fat. If you imagine your fat as a brick wall, lipase is a chisel that removes the bricks one by one. The bricks are now free to travel, to be used around the body and also burned up for energy.

Lipase needs water in good supply to work well. Very simplistically, this is how it works:

$$Fat + Water + Lipase = Fatty Acids$$

Fatty acids are the small building blocks of fat. They are like the bricks in the wall. Fatty acids are small enough to be released into your circulation and will be picked up by cells around your body needing energy. The more fatty acids released from your fat, the slimmer you become. They are released easier when you are well hydrated.

The Bottom Line

If you're not drinking enough water on an everyday basis you're likely to eat more than you need, in order to satisfy your 'hunger' (which is actually thirst). Your body needs far more water than it does food. It goes without saying - the more you eat, unless you're very active, the fatter you will get. At the very least, you'll struggle to lose weight.

So water has three direct effects to help you with your fat loss, and keep it off:

1. Water provides calorie-free hydroelectric energy to your brain
2. Water's abundant presence is necessary for lipase to work efficiently when breaking down your fat
3. When your body is well hydrated any hunger you feel is genuinely for food and not water

Hydrating yourself properly, if you're not doing it already, will start to tip the scales in your favour.

How To Get The Best From Water

As a general rule of thumb you should aim for about 8 glasses of water a day. Maybe a little less if you're petite, and more if you're a really big person. 8 glasses is about 4 pints, or just over 2 litres.

If you're not used to drinking much water, follow this guide to get you started:

- Have a glass or two first thing in the morning. This is the most important time to hydrate; you'll be dehydrated because you haven't had a drink all night (you lose water every time you breathe out - this adds up a lot overnight!)
- Drink water regularly during the day
- Have a glass 15-30 minutes before food – you will then be satisfying genuine hunger when you eat and not thirst

- Dehydrating drinks, like caffeine and alcohol, drain water from your body and the consequence is that the activity of lipase is reduced, AND you'll feel more 'hungry' than you should, which will make you inclined to eat more.

You'll find out more about caffeine and alcohol later, but just bear in mind they're not helping you. That's not to say you have to give them up, so don't panic!

What If You Don't Like Water?

Think for a minute about what your ancestors used to drink. There was only water. If you can really say that you don't like water very much, consider how far removed you must be from what is good and natural for your body. Think about that for a moment - how has this happened?

If you're like most people you'll drink at least one of these three things: tea, coffee or alcohol. Did you like any of these as a child? I doubt it. I certainly didn't but I managed to change easily enough. And you learned to like them too, because you kept trying them. You kept trying because you wanted to like them. You can do the same here and learn to enjoy water again. You might even want to add it as one of your steps.

A woman on my course wasn't used to drinking so

much water and kept forgetting. Her idea to overcome this was to start the day with eight pennies in one pocket. Just having them there reminded her to drink water through the day. As she finished a glass she would move a penny to the opposite pocket. When you do something like this for long enough you eventually establish a new habit and just do it automatically; you won't always need reminders.

What could you do to remind yourself to drink more water?

What About Alternatives?

Okay, I admit it. I don't exclusively drink water because I like a bit of variety. While water is best, these are some healthy variations:

- Hot or cold water with a squeeze of fresh lime or lemon juice
- Or, try some fresh mint leaves or other herbs if you have some in your garden – again, in hot or cold water
- Caffeine-free herbal teas.
- Sparkling water

Beware of cordials and squash. They will either be full of sugar, or if sugar-free, they'll be sweetened with artificial chemical sweeteners like aspartame, saccharin or sucralose (these are commonly used). Artificial sweeteners were developed in labs by chemists. Aspartame, in particular, is linked to a long list of health problems, including obesity.

Calorie-free soft drinks can add to your weight problems because of the artificial sweeteners that have chemical effects on your brain – avoid them like the plague! Chemicals that aren't natural and which shouldn't be in your body do weird things to you – none of them good.

On my online course I introduce people to water in the first week, and for those who take the message on board, it doesn't take long to start feeling the benefits. Here's feedback I got from Jacqueline:

'My old routine was to get out of bed and have a mug of tea, swiftly followed by another, and then a third and fourth mug as soon as I got to work. I needed this to wake me up and 'kick start' me before I could face the day, or so I thought. Instead of drinking tea the moment my eyes open, I've started drinking a pint of water as soon as I wake up. I can't describe what a difference it's made to me. Instead of craving cuppa after cuppa, I find I'm not thirsty after my pint of water. And I find it slips down so easily, which makes me realise how dehydrated I must be every morning (I'm talking about the ordinary days when I haven't been boozing the night before). It's hard to believe that something as simple as drinking a big glass of water first thing can make me feel so energised, but it does.

*I'm still drinking tea, but just find I'm not desperate
for it any more. I'm drinking 8 glasses of water a day
now and I just feel so good! This is the first change
I've made so far, and I'm still astounded at what a
difference something so simple and easy can make.*

Proper hydration is going to make fat loss a lot easier
for you - I would suggest this is an essential part of
your plan. Have you put it in your plan yet? How are
you going to make sure you incorporate this in your
everyday life?

The next thing we're going to look at is other,
seemingly small things, which are essential for
efficient fat loss.

13. Your Tiny Helpers – The Essential Nutrients

Before I get into this section I want to share with you
the results of some fascinating research. Normally,
I find animal experiments distasteful, but this one
caught my interest. This information came from a
book written in 1978: Goldot by Lewis E, Cook Jr. and
Junko Yasui.

A number of rats were split into three groups with
the aim of feeding them differently and observing the
effects. This was to be done over the course of the
rat's lifetime, the equivalent of eighty human years.

The rats were then put to sleep and their bodies studied to see what shape they were in.

Rats are a bit like humans, in that they'll eat anything available, which might be one reason why they were chosen for the experiment.

Group one was fed on a 'junk food' diet filled with refined, processed and pre-made food. They were also given vitamins and medicine. This was comparable to a typical western diet. There wasn't any raw or wholefoods fed to this group. Unfortunately, none of these rats reached the target age; they all succumbed to disease before reaching it.

As they died, their bodies were examined to see what had killed them. It was noted that the rats were all fat. Looking closer at their insides, it became apparent that a large quantity had died of vascular diseases, i.e. heart problems and strokes. Many others had died of cancer.

In addition to their disastrous state of health these rats kept getting ill with minor illnesses throughout their lives, like colds and chest infections. They developed things like cataracts and arthritis. Their emotional health appeared unstable and they kept attacking each other. So, although they were alive, they weren't living happy or healthy lives.

Group two was fed only on raw and wholefood, food that had not been processed or refined in any way. You could look at this food and see exactly what it was – nothing was added and nothing taken away.

This group all reached their target age, the human equivalent of eighty years-old. They all had a normal body weight, none were fat. They were put down and their bodies examined.

These rats had no evidence of any vascular disease, i.e. no impending heart attacks or strokes. They had no tumours or cancer. In fact these 'old' rats had bodies comparable to young rats.

In addition to being disease free these rats didn't get many minor infections; they obviously had great immune systems. They didn't get cataracts or suffer with arthritis. They appeared happy and playful, and displayed very little aggression towards each other.

Group three is the one that caught my interest the most. This group was fed the junk diet until they reached the human equivalent of forty years of age. Fortunately, they all made it to this age, although they weren't a happy bunch – they were fat and aggressive towards each other and they kept getting minor illnesses. But then they were switched to the wholefood diet.

Not only did they all reach the target age, they all lost weight too, and quickly. Behavioural problems settled and minor health problems cleared up. When they were put down their bodies were examined and found to be in the same great shape as group two, i.e. as if they'd been eating raw and wholefoods all their lives.

The rats that started out on 'junk food' had their health and weight turned around completely by the switch to healthy wholefoods. Any damage done was reversed by their wholesome diet. The weight gain was also reversed and they regained a normal healthy weight without excess fat. They became happier rats, interacting with each other in playful, non-aggressive ways.

I know these are rats are not people but this really gives food for thought, doesn't it? There's plenty of evidence that humans can reverse some illnesses and disease by eating food that's good for them, and avoiding what isn't. In fact, a minority of doctors, and lots of 'alternative' health practitioners, approach illness with diet change, not pills.

One of the problems with a junk food diet is that it is deficient of nutrients essential to your health.

What Are Essential Nutrients?

There are a number of things that are absolutely essential to your health. Without them, you'll become ill and die at some point. Essential nutrients are:

- 21 Minerals, including:
  - Iron – needed to transport oxygen around your body
  - Magnesium – important in energy production within your body
  - Calcium – essential for strong bones and teeth
  - Zinc – vital for a healthy immune system
  - Iodine – essential for your thyroid gland, and hence necessary for a healthy metabolism
  - Selenium – essential ingredient used in the process of releasing energy from glucose and fatty acids
- 13 Vitamins, including:
  - Vitamin A – vital for a healthy immune system
  - B vitamins – needed for a healthy nervous system and brain
  - Vitamin C – important for the health of your heart
  - Vitamin D – plays a protective role against cancer
- 8 Amino acids – the small building blocks of protein
- 2 Essential fatty acids – more coming up about these later
- A source of energy – i.e. calories

- Water
- Oxygen
- Sunshine – your biggest source of vitamin D

There are many other things needed for good health too, but you don't need to know all the details. That's because, when you eat well, you naturally get them all. Humans eating primitive (i.e. healthy) diets don't worry about vitamins and minerals, they don't need to. They eat wholesome, nutritious foods, so all the above is included with their diet. When you eat well you generally get enough vitamins, minerals, essential amino acids and fats, and, of course, energy.

You already know about how important water is. Oxygen is obviously vital, everyone knows that. But did you know cancer thrives in oxygen-poor states? This makes exercise relevant not only to your fat loss efforts but also to your health in general. When you exercise you oxygenate your whole body. Through deep breathing and muscle contractions oxygen-rich blood is pumped all around your body, bringing life and vitality to every part of you.

When you hardly ever exercise your blood flow can get sluggish and slow, resulting in oxygen levels not being optimum in some parts of your body for significant lengths of time. This is because you're only breathing shallowly, so only taking in a bare minimum of oxygen. If your muscles aren't being used much, you aren't pumping oxygen-rich blood throughout your body. In the couch potato some areas of the body can end up oxygen deprived, setting the scene for disease.

This is why people who exercise regularly are at less risk of cancer (as well as being thinner). There is much more coming up about exercise in part four.

Why Are Essential Nutrients Relevant To Fat Loss?

You already know that water is a vital ingredient needed to break fat down. Vitamins and minerals are needed too.

To help me explain, imagine you're going to light a real fire, an open fire, or one in a log burner. You need to get a few things ready. You've got screwed-up newspaper at the bottom with kindling wood on top. You've got heavier wood ready for when the fire gets going, and perhaps some coal too. Basically, you've got a lot of energy ready to burn:

- Paper
- Kindling wood
- Bigger wood
- Coal

But at present it's sat there doing nothing. You have to light it to release the energy. You pick up a box of matches, take one out and go to strike the match. That's when you notice the scratchy bit on the side of the box is missing. On the face of it you've got everything to have a nice warm fire, but you're stuck.

Your other option is to take a couple of bits of wood and rub them together until you get a spark big enough to light your fire. You'll get there in the end doing it this way, but it's going to take you a while.

Paper, kindling, wood, coal + *functioning matchbox* =
Fast energy release
Paper, kindling, wood, coal + *what else can we use?* =
Slow energy release

Let's get back to your body, where the essential nutrients are very much like the rough bit on the packet of matches.

Your body needs a good supply of essential nutrients to burn fat, to release its energy and make you slimmer. If you're not eating nutritious food on a regular basis you won't have a good supply of these. So when your body attempts to burn your fat it can see it's got loads of stored energy (like the wood and coal), but when it goes to burn it, some necessary ingredients are missing. It's just like missing the scratchy bit on the matchbox.

Fortunately, your body is clever so it will find another way. But the same as rubbing sticks together takes a long time, so does burning your body fat if you haven't got plenty of essential nutrients to kick-start the process.

This:
Fatty acids + oxygen + *essential nutrients* = Fast energy release (and you getting slimmer)
is much better than this:
Fatty acids + oxygen + *what else can we use?* = Slow energy release (and your fat taking much longer to shed)

Regarding the food you eat today - if your body isn't given everything it needs to burn the calories you're eating (i.e. if they're not included in the food), and you don't have a good store of them already, these calories are far more likely to be stored as fat.

A diet high in refined food will be deficient of the small nutrients. If your diet is running low on these, even a modest calorie intake can cause problems with your weight.

The other problem with not getting enough of these essential nutrients is that your body still needs them for a whole host of other reasons. Your blood still needs iron and your thyroid still needs iodine. You may be taking in an excess of calories but you can still be malnourished if you haven't got enough of the essential nutrients. Because your body still needs them it will try and get you to eat more, in an attempt to get the things it's lacking, so you feel hungry even though you don't need calories.

Malnourishment, due to eating lots of refined and processed food, leads to deficiencies of the essential nutrients. This leads to your appetite being ramped up in your body's attempt to get you to feed it some real nourishment. This can cause cravings and hunger, even though you don't need any more calories. What you need is essential nutrients and good nourishment.

The message here is that you need nutritious food on a regular basis to efficiently burn your fat and curb your hunger. Examples of nutritious foods are coming up.

Why Are Many People Deficient Of Essential Nutrients?

It comes down to the quality of the food you eat, and by that I mean, how nutritious it is. Nutritious food is packed full of essential nutrients, as well as calories. Remember, you need the essential nutrients to burn the calories efficiently.

Much of today's westernised food has been refined. For example, flour is refined and turned from wholegrain to white flour. This gives it a finer texture and a longer shelf life. During the refining process much of the nutritious goodness is removed from the grain; this is because the bran and germ of the wholegrain are taken away. When these are removed much of the nutrition goes with them:

Nutrient	% Lost Due To Refining
Calcium	60
Iron	76
Magnesium	85
Potassium	77
Zinc	78
B vitamins	72-81
Vitamin E	86
Essential Fatty Acids	95
Protein	33
Fibre	95

These figures are taken from work done by Henry A. Schroeder in the U.S.

Whenever you eat refined white stuff you're eating nutritionally deficient food. This includes anything made out of white flour: white bread, most cakes, biscuits and pastries; white pasta. The same is true for white rice, most of the nutrition has been removed yet most of the calories are left behind.

Anything that has been refined and gone from wholegrain to white and refined is just a whole load of calories without the vitamins and minerals needed by your body to burn it.

When you compare that to something that's been left in its natural form, i.e. wholegrain, you have everything that Mother Nature put there. As well as the calories you have the smaller nutrients your body needs to light the fire and burn them off. You also still have the fibre.

Food that contains fibre fills you up quicker than white, refined stuff. There's only so much you can fit in your stomach in one go. With white, refined food you can eat until your stomach is filled entirely with calories. When you eat whole foods you're filling your stomach with fibre as well as calories, so you consume fewer calories.

Can you eat a small doughnut in one go? Of course you can. Will you have room for another? Quite possibly, especially if you like doughnuts. Can you eat ten carrots in one go? Probably, but it's going to take a lot longer and you'll probably get quite full. Could you then eat another ten?

One doughnut has roughly the same amount of calories as ten carrots. Refined food, like a doughnut, makes it VERY easy to eat a lot of calories. There's no fibre to fill you up. There's also precious little in the way of nutrients, so you're relying on other nutritious food to get the smaller nutrients and burn these calories up. It's not so easy to eat a lot of calories when you eat real food; the fibre makes it difficult.

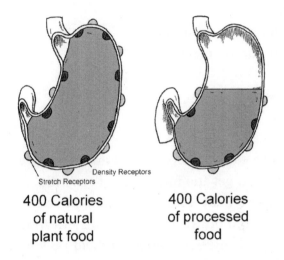

Density Receptors
Stretch Receptors

400 Calories of natural plant food

400 Calories of processed food

I've noticed a big difference in the amount of rice I eat when I'm at a friend's and served white rice, compared to the wholegrain I eat at home. I have to eat so much more of the white to feel full. At the same time, I've had to consume many more calories to get to the same level of fullness. This is the difference fibre makes.

How To Get More Essential Nutrients

Obviously choose real foods, in their natural state, over refined, man-made, nutritionally deficient 'food'.

Examples of real food include:
• Fruit

- Vegetables
- Wholegrain cereals – rice, spelt (a type of wheat), rye
- Good quality fresh fish
- Good quality meat
- Eggs
- Seeds
- Nuts

It's good to eat a variety of food and it's one way of ensuring you get the full range of essential nutrients. As long as you eat a range of real food you will get what you need on the essential nutrient front, without having to be concerned about individual vitamins or minerals. Mother Nature has put everything you need into the food you're designed to eat. By variety, I mean different varieties of fruit and veg (don't stick to the same ones all the time), a variety of seed and nuts, and several different types of fish and meat.

Some people have said to me, 'But I don't like wholegrain rice and/or bread'.

In the water chapter I explained how you can learn to like new things. The same applies here. Keep trying the healthier options and have them more often. What happens with most people is they get to the stage where they quite like the wholegrain versions. Eventually, they really like them, and might not even bother with the white, refined stuff, or if they do, they just have it as an occasional indulgence.

Remember, the real food helps you burn fat and lose weight. The refined food makes you fat. Bearing this in mind may help steer your taste buds in a different direction. And there's no rush, do this bit by bit.

As you progress through this book you'll learn more and more about how to make your food more health friendly, i.e. how to eat with good nutrition in mind. But here are a few things to get you thinking:

- Raw foods retain their essential nutrients – fruit and salads are great
- Cooking destroys many essential nutrients
- Different types of cooking destroy more nutrients than others

Different cooking methods have a vastly different effect on the end product, in terms of the essential nutrients left at the point of consuming. It's surprising just how much is lost when you microwave food.

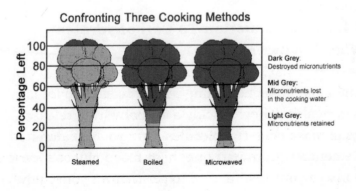

Confronting Three Cooking Methods

Dark Grey:
Destroyed micronutrients

Mid Grey:
Micronutrients lost in the cooking water

Light Grey:
Micronutrients retained

The thing to take away from this is, if you're starting with a healthy and nutritious piece of food, steam it, if possible, to retain the goodness. You will obliterate the nutrition by putting it in the microwave.

If you're boiling vegetables to cook them, a lot of the nutrients will be lost in the water. If you're using that water as part of soup or gravy you're making, that's okay. Otherwise, a lot of the smaller nutrients will be lost. Perhaps you could begin to steam your veg instead?

Other great ways to get plenty of essential nutrients is to have smoothies and fresh, homemade fruit and vegetable juices. You'll find some ideas and recipes towards the end of the book.

Your next BIG win when it comes to fat loss is getting to grips with the carbs you eat. There are massive gains to be made once you understand what's going on.

14. An Introduction To Carbohydrates
What Is A Carbohydrate?

The most important thing when it comes to fat loss and health is how quickly a carbohydrate releases its glucose (sugar) molecules after you've eaten it. Remember, from part one: high blood glucose levels damage your health, and to get it down your body converts it to fat.

Going back to the wall analogy I used with fat, a similar thing goes on with carbohydrates. In their stuck-together, complete form (like a wall) they appear as things like bread, potatoes, breakfast cereals and rice. In their broken down form they're largely glucose.

When carbs are broken down into their building blocks you end up with a load of glucose molecules (isolated bricks that are not part of a wall anymore).

When you eat a carbohydrate your body has to absorb it from your intestines. It can't absorb a 'brick wall', it's just too big, and it therefore has to break the brick wall down into building blocks. Glucose molecules are very small, small enough to travel across your intestinal wall and into your bloodstream.

The most important thing about carbs is how quickly the 'wall' is broken down into its bricks, i.e. how fast the glucose molecules are released. This is very relevant to your fat loss efforts and you'll find out why shortly.

The Glycaemic Index

An indication to the speed at which carbs are broken down and absorbed is given by their number on the glycaemic index (GI).

Glucose was given the GI of 100. This was worked out by giving people a glucose drink and testing their blood sugar level afterwards. Years ago researchers fed people all sorts of foods and recorded the change in their blood sugar, and compared it to the reference point of glucose. All other carbs are compared to glucose and scored accordingly. You do not need to know much about the GI of most foods. Broad principles are all you need to improve your health and fat loss.

Obviously, if you take in pure glucose, it doesn't need any breaking down. It travels straight across your gut wall and into your bloodstream, pushing your blood sugar up very quickly.

Carbs that push your blood sugar up fast and high (like refined white rice, which has a high GI at 89) force your body to deal with a high glucose situation. It does this by laying down fat.

Why Is The Glycaemic Index So Relevant?

Generally speaking, your blood sugar is tightly controlled within a narrow margin. It needs to be high enough for you to function, but becomes very bad for you when it gets too high. I touched on this in part one and will be revisiting this issue later in the book.

When you eat food that causes your blood sugar to

rise, your body reacts to bring it down to protect itself. It does this by producing insulin. Insulin is secreted by your pancreas into your bloodstream.

Insulin brings your blood sugar down to normal, but how does it do that? There are two storehouses for excess glucose. By excess, I mean that which is above what you're currently using for energy expenditure.

The first storehouse is your glycogen stores, which are mainly found in your liver and muscles. When the glucose is stored here, it's easy to get back out, and it comes back out as it went in – as glucose. This is partly what keeps you going in between meals. There is only limited capacity here, so once your glycogen stores are full, the rest of the glucose has to go to the second storehouse.

Your second storehouse is your fat cells. You have practically limitless storage capacity here. When you eat more glucose than you're using and can store as glycogen, it gets sucked up by your fat cells. It is also converted to fat; it's no longer glucose. This means it's not readily available like it would have been in your glycogen stores.

The general rule of thumb is that whenever you eat something that causes insulin to be secreted you'll be laying down fat. Some carbs cause your body to produce a lot more insulin than others. A lot more insulin means a lot more fat formation.

The quicker a carbohydrate is broken down into its glucose molecules the quicker your blood sugar will rise. This produces a corresponding rise in insulin as it chases the blood sugar up in an effort to get it down. The higher the glucose rise, the higher the insulin rise.

This graph shows what happens to your blood glucose when you eat two different types of carbohydrates. They're both eaten at a time when the body's blood glucose is at a normal level. One of these is broken down fast and the other much slower. These two foods may have had the same amount of calories, but they have very different effects on your body. They could represent white rice compared to wholegrain rice.

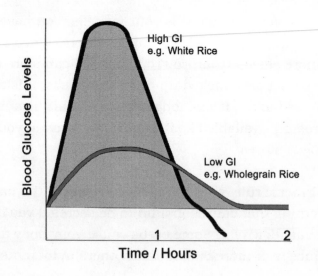

White rice has been refined and it's no longer
a natural food; much of its goodness has been
stripped away and what's left is pretty much pure
carbohydrate (i.e. calories). Because things like
protein and most of the fibre has gone, there isn't
much holding the contents of the rice together. So
when it hits your stomach there's very little holding
the 'wall' together. It literally falls apart the moment
it hits your stomach, and the glucose molecules are
released rapidly, very much like cutting the string on
a beaded necklace.

The glucose is released very fast, and consequently,
your blood sugar goes up very quickly.

The GI of white rice is around 89; this is not much
lower than pure glucose. It's almost like eating
spoonfuls of glucose. (White basmati rice is lower,
at 67).

Because high glucose levels are harmful to your body,
it responds robustly and quickly by releasing a large
amount of insulin. Remember: the more insulin you
have floating around, the more fat you're laying down.

Compare this to what happens with a natural
wholefood like wholegrain rice, which is still intact.
Not only does it retain its essential nutrients but it
also has its fibre and full protein content. This makes
a wholegrain carbohydrate like a solid brick wall as

far as digestion is concerned. It takes longer for your digestive system to break down. Consequently, the glucose release is slower and gentler. This gives you a chance to burn off some of the glucose as you're going about your day (meaning less for storage). It also means your insulin response is much less. This means less fat being laid down.

The GI for wholegrain basmati rice is 50 – what a difference!

The GI range is as follows:
- Low GI – 55 or less
- Medium GI - 56-69
- High GI – 70 and over

But there's something else relevant here too. Because your body views high blood glucose as an emergency that needs to be dealt with immediately, its reaction can overshoot the mark. You can see with the white rice example the blood sugar actually ends up below normal range. This is important, because when you're in this state you tend to feel ravenously hungry.

Compare that to the wholegrain rice. The blood glucose gradually comes back to normal and at some point you will start to feel peckish. Remember, you could have eaten the same amount of calories with these two choices, but one will keep you going for longer than the other. However, in everyday life, the likelihood is you'd have eaten more white than brown rice, because it takes more of the white to fill you up.

Can you see the damage that's done to food when it's refined?

This damage is passed onto you when you eat it.

Can you see why some carbs are a lot more fattening than others?

The worst sort of carbs:
* Don't fill you up in the first place, so you end up eating more
* Cause insulin spikes that lead to fat lay down
* Cause low blood sugar, which makes you eat more

When it comes to health and your weight, refined carbs and sugar have nothing positive going for them. Here are some examples of high, medium and low GI common breakfast choices:
* High
  * Cornflakes 80
  * Coco-pops 77
  * Cheerios 74
  * Special K 69
* Medium
  * Porridge 55
* Low
  * Natural wholegrain muesli 40

- All-bran 50

Notice that all the refined ones - the ones you wouldn't have a clue what they were made of without looking at the ingredients - have a high GI. The less grains are 'interfered with', the lower their GI tends to be. Natural food is much better for you.

Did Our Ancestors Eat Carbohydrates?

It's worth bearing in mind that it's only within the last 10,000 years or so, i.e. since agriculture became prevalent, that the diet of human beings contained so much carbohydrate. Before this time, humans ate very little in the way of grain, e.g. wheat and rice.

Before agriculture, carbohydrates in the human diet came largely from fruit and vegetables. So we can assume that these are healthy things to eat. Our ancestors, like modern day hunter-gatherers, would have had very low levels of insulin, due to a low-carb diet. This is one of the reasons they were, and still are, slim.

A high carbohydrate diet is not a particularly natural diet for a human to eat. Even choosing carbs with a low GI stimulates insulin secretion. For this reason, you'll lose more fat if you keep your carb portions small and eat more of other things. I do this by always having a big serving of steamed veg or salad when I'm eating carbs. This helps to fill me up so I don't need to eat a great plateful of carbs to feel satisfied.

Some people eat very high carb diets, something easy to do with a typical western diet. You could have cereal or toast for breakfast, a sandwich for lunch and pasta or potatoes with your main meal. This is a lot of carbs in a day, which all cause insulin to be released. Obviously, you can minimise that by choosing whole grains, but even better is reducing the carbs you consume by eating more of other things.

I will give you some ideas at the end of the book, but to give you an idea: you could have a smoothie for breakfast, an omelette for lunch, and for your main meal, you could have a piece of fish with loads of steamed veg and a couple of boiled potatoes (with butter – yes, I said butter! You'll find out more about that later). This daily menu features fewer carbs, which means less insulin production and less fat subsequently laid down.

15. Wheat Is Not Your Friend

Wheat has undergone huge genetic manipulation over the last fifty years or so. This was originally driven by the need to feed more people.

First of all, food producers wanted to increase the yield of the wheat, so its genetic material was manipulated to produce more crop and bigger grains within each plant. This caused a problem, because wheat is a grass, and as such, gets quite tall when it goes to seed. With oversized grains at the top, stems would buckle under the weight.

This problem was solved genetically, by changing the wheat plant's stature so that it was much shorter. The modern-day wheat plant is only about a foot tall; it's a dwarf compared to its ancestor. This also makes it much easier to harvest.

In addition to these changes, wheat has been genetically changed to produce plants that are resistant to drought, resistant to various diseases and tough enough to withstand a variety of pesticides and chemical fertilisers. Further genetic change has been made to produce a variety of different flours suitable for different styles of cooking. You wouldn't use strong bread flour if you wanted to make a light, fluffy cake, for example, it just wouldn't work.

So genetic change was engineered for this reason, that reason and the other reason. But... has anyone checked if the end product is still okay to eat? Not really. Is it okay to eat? Well, let's see.

Wheat: The 'Healthy' Whole Grain

In the '80s there was a drive to get people to switch

from refined food to whole grains, so that they were healthier. A significant amount of people shifted from things like white bread and rice to wholegrain and rates of heart disease and cancer improved, for a short time. This will have been because of the increased amounts of essential nutrients in whole grains.

As a general rule, you would expect the wholegrain version of a grain to have a significantly lower GI than its white refined counterpart, as demonstrated by rice. It would be reasonable to expect the same with white bread when compared with wholegrain, wouldn't it?

A carb's GI number reflects how quickly it releases its glucose when you eat it. The lower the better when it comes to carbs like bread, rice, breakfast cereals and snacks.

Spelt is a type of wheat. It's an ancient relative of modern day wheat that hasn't gone through the significant genetic change that conventional wheat has (the type most commonly found on our supermarket shelves). It was widely grown by the Romans. The gluten (a protein occurring in many grains) in spelt is easily digested (unlike that found in modern day wheat).

Bread made out of white, refined spelt flour has a GI of 70. This is high, which means the sugar is released fast, just like white rice. Wholegrain spelt bread comes in at around 54. This is an awful lot better for you.

Conventional mass-produced wheat is what the vast majority of bread and breakfast cereals are made with. Bread made out of white, refined wheat flour has a GI of 70, which is what you would expect. What is surprising is that many wholegrain versions of conventional wheat bread also have a GI as high as 70. So, although you're getting the benefit of the extra nutrients with wholegrain bread, it isn't healthier when it comes to your weight.

What about other commonly eaten wheat products, like healthy wholegrain breakfast cereals such as Shredded Wheat? This has a GI of 67, which is quite high and means it will produce a significant insulin splurge that will result in you laying fat down. So much for healthy!

Shredded Wheat is obviously better than something like sugary jam on white toast, because it still has its essential nutrients. However, if you're concerned about your weight, there are better choices e.g. toast made out of spelt. Even better would be to have breakfast that wasn't based on grains e.g. an omelette.

What things do you commonly eat that has 'normal' wheat in? There are quite a few potentials: bread, breakfast cereals, cakes, biscuits, pastries, crackers, crisp-breads, snacks. You'll also find wheat in nearly all ready-made and processed food.

Wheat So Far

So far you've learnt that things made with either white or wholegrain wheat flour tend to have a high GI. The white version of any grain is guaranteed to make the GI high. The wholegrain version does not necessarily mean it will be lower, however, when it comes to modern day conventional wheat.

A high GI means high insulin. High insulin means fat lay down. Also remember that whenever insulin is present your body can't break any fat down. High insulin has the subsequent effect of causing low blood sugar. This will ramp up your appetite.

I'm afraid it gets worse for modern conventional wheat.

More About Wheat

Endorphins are messengers released by certain cells in your brain. They're released when you do things like get into a warm bath, give your dog or your cat a cuddle, when you exercise, when you've had a good giggle with a friend, or from watching your children play. You feel the effect of endorphins when they attach to endorphin receptors on other cells in your brain. This is like putting a key into a lock. When the receptor has been filled, you feel good.

On the dark side, this is what happens with heroin. Heroin and morphine are very similar to our natural endorphins, and as such, attach to the receptors – providing that temporary 'feel good' feeling. But, obviously, this feeling is short-lived, and there are far more downsides to using heroin than this short term good feeling. When users 'come down' from this feeling they're left feeling low and craving the pleasant feelings again, driving them to use more heroin.

Genetically-altered protein (gluten) in wheat has the ability to attach to your endorphin receptors. This gluten should break down into its constituent amino acids before reaching the bloodstream but genetically-manipulated gluten is difficult to digest, and in some people, manages to get across the gut wall without being fully broken down. In other grains, like spelt, the gluten is easily digested and gets broken down properly before being absorbed.

If gluten gets into your bloodstream without being properly broken down, it can attach to your endorphin receptors. This will make you feel good, or help pick you up from a low. You don't feel so good when this wears off, which can lead you, unconsciously, to need another hit. This will feel like a craving for wheat-based food.

On another level this is exactly what happens with heroin.

If you've ever felt like your eating is out of control, and you eat wheat on a regular basis, this might be a reason.

Some people are more prone to this effect than others. It's a bit like alcohol. Alcohol is an addictive substance, but not everyone who drinks becomes addicted or has a problem with it. It's the same with wheat.

So, if you eat wheat regularly, like a lot of people do, this is potentially very bad news for your weight because it drives your appetite by:

- Causing low blood sugar, because of high insulin release
- Causing addiction, from the effect of genetically altered proteins on your brain

Eating wheat regularly can leave you in a situation where you feel out of control with regards to your eating, where you can't lose weight, or you're putting weight on.

Pasta Is Different

Here's some good news, at least.

Durum wheat, which is used to make pasta and couscous, hasn't gone through the same degree of extensive genetic manipulation that other wheat has. The gluten is easier to digest, so addiction due to altered gluten is less likely.

The GI of pasta is a lot better than bread made from conventional wheat:
- GI of white spaghetti = 58 (medium GI)
- GI of wholegrain spaghetti = 42 (low GI)

Obviously, the wholegrain version is better, in terms of its lower GI. It will also retain its essential nutrients. White pasta will have lost these.

Couscous is made from white, refined durum wheat, so this too will have lost most of its essential nutrients, and is therefore not really a wise choice. If you like couscous, try the wholegrain quinoa in its place. Quinoa is a small grain; at first glance, you might think it's couscous, but it's so much better – it's packed with essential nutrients and its GI is lower. You can find quinoa in most supermarkets.

16. Changes To Make With Carbs

When you get your carbs right you stand to lose significant body fat. When you reduce refined white carbs (and things made from them) as much as possible you'll turbo-charge your fat loss. Refined white carbs include all white flours, white rice and sugar.

Pay attention to how much sugar you have. Refined white sugar has no essential nutrients at all. It's purely calories and doesn't contain the essential ingredients to burn its own calories. It's like a huge pile of wood and coal without a matchbox. It's in nearly all pre-made and processed foods, sometimes by the bucket load. If food needs a label it probably has sugar in it, and is, therefore, not going to be very good for your waistline.

Refined white sugar is completely unnecessary and alien to a natural human diet. Whenever you have food or drinks with sugar your body makes insulin and you will lay down fat. Low fat, processed foods often have a lot of sugar and/or refined white carbs added to them. This is to replace flavour and substance lost by removing the fat. More on this later.

Things to cut back on as much as possible:
- White flour, and all things made from it
  - Bread
  - Cakes

- Biscuits
- Croissants
- Pastry
- Crisp-breads
- Sugar
- White rice

A quick reminder why it's a good idea to cut back on these:

- They shoot your blood glucose up, which causes a surge in insulin release and fat lay down
- The surge of insulin creates a rebound low blood sugar that makes you very hungry soon after
- They've lost their essential nutrients so leave you malnourished, which also drives your appetite
- They've lost their fibre resulting in you eating more to feel full

If you eat a lot of refined white carbs, gradually change these to wholegrain versions. Whole grains are slow release, meaning the glucose in them is released gradually. This gives you a chance to burn the energy off as it travels through your body. Your glycogen stores are less likely to be overwhelmed and have a chance of coping before your fat cells take over. Your insulin response will be significantly less so there's less fat laid down.

Even with these better choices, it's not a good idea to have a great big plateful of them in one go. This is because, ultimately, the glucose has to be dealt with. If you overdo it here the glucose will still be destined for fat conversion, but it's more difficult to overdo it with whole grains because they fill you up more quickly. Having a big serving of vegetables or salad helps fill you up too, as well as feed your body lots of vitamins and minerals.

Examples of better carbs to eat:
- Wholegrain rice, particularly basmati, due to its low GI
- Wholegrain flour (more on this in the next section)
- Quinoa - a grain that can be used in the same way as couscous
- Pulses, like lentils, beans, peas

Another commonly eaten carb is the potato. The news is not good here if you're a potato lover, I'm afraid.

Potatoes have a very high GI, e.g. chips are around 75 on the index and mashed potatoes are a whopping 82. This is really, really high. The glucose in potatoes is released very fast indeed, shooting your blood sugar up very quickly.

There's no need to stop eating them, just go easy on how many in one setting. For example, when I have boiled potatoes I only tend to have two or three little ones. You can bring the GI down a bit by eating the skins too. The skins give your digestion a bit more work to do and this slows the glucose rush down a little.

Consider Four Weeks Without Wheat

This suggestion usually raises some eyebrows! First of all, there's no need to rush into this. If you're like most people you might be eating wheat once, twice, or even three times a day. So, this is going to take some thought before you do it.

Studies have shown that when people cut wheat out of their diet they eat 250-450 fewer calories per day. That would add up to an awful lot of calories over a year. This is why people who seriously cut down on their wheat intake generally lose weight (providing they don't eat white, refined substitutes), and often do it quite quickly.

Why do people eat significantly fewer calories when they stop eating wheat? For starters, they aren't having massive spikes of insulin, and subsequent rebound low blood sugar (causing ravenous hunger). Because of less insulin there's less fat lay down. Also, the abnormal proteins in genetically-manipulated wheat are no longer stimulating endorphin receptors in the brain. This again reduces appetite.

Towards the back of the book, you'll find some ideas to get you going, but bread seems to be people's biggest stumbling block. To continue enjoying bread, switch to spelt, you might not even notice a difference. Rye is another option but this is quite different and more of an acquired taste. I think it should go without saying by now that the best choice is wholegrain, NOT white. Both of these grains have a lower GI and their gluten is easier to digest.

Depending where you shop, you might struggle to get spelt bread; if this is the case, consider looking further afield. Some supermarkets do sell both spelt and rye, others don't. You should get some in quality bakeries - another place is health food shops. You really can't beat, however, homemade bread, and you'll find a recipe at the end of the book for a spelt loaf. It's easier than you may think.

Many people find other benefits to ditching wheat too. Top of the list is greatly improved (often eliminated) irritable bowel syndrome (IBS) symptoms. People also have flatter stomachs because they're not bloated and many notice that their energy levels rise. General aches and pains, and arthritic pain, can improve. Some people have told me that ditching wheat got rid of their heartburn.

I suggest trialling no wheat for four weeks. See what happens, see how you feel and then make a decision about continuing or not. You're not going to know how good you could feel without trying it. As I keep reminding you, though – there's no rush. Don't make things difficult for yourself. Do one thing at a time and you'll get there.

Another Health Implication From Too Many Carbs

The following is a blog entry I wrote in June 2013:

Sugar and cancer

If you eat a lot of sugar, and/or foods that are converted to sugar, you may be increasing your chances of getting cancer. If you already have cancer you may be speeding up its progression by continuing to eat sugar.

This is another good reason to get your carbs right. Last week we had an introduction to foods with good carbs, in relation to weight. Food isn't only about weight. Our regular eating habits can have more dire consequences than piling on the pounds. It's usually weight that takes centre stage, though.

Many cancers, particularly the common ones, happen more often to people who are overweight. Poor dietary choices aren't exclusive to the overweight by any means, and obviously slim people do get cancer too.

Otto Heinrich Warburg won two Nobel Prizes in the first half of the 20th century. He linked the breakdown of sugar in our bodies as the prime cause, and ongoing supporter, of cancer. I find it amazing that this knowledge has been available to us for nearly a hundred years, but that in that time our consumption of sugar, and foods that turn into sugar when we eat them, has increased dramatically.

People recognise that something has gone wrong with their eating when they get fat. Often the first thing they do is attempt to change what they eat. Unfortunately, this often involves going on a diet rather than learning about what your body needs to be fit and slim.

What I find surprising is that when people get something awful, like cancer, very little focus is put on diet. This is probably because doctors rarely bring it up. We doctors learned next to nothing about nutrition at medical school, maybe that's why.

The human body does not need sugar and refined, white carbohydrates. To be healthy, reduce your sugar intake to a minimum and choose whole grain over refined, white rubbish that turns to sugar almost as soon as it hits your stomach.

This is yet another very good reason to look at what you're doing in terms of the carbs you're eating on a regular basis. Remember, it's what you do most of the time that counts.

17. An Insight Into The Food Industry

The most important thing to know about the food industry is what it cares for most, and that isn't you. In fact, you're probably being manipulated every time you go food shopping.

The food industry is BIG business, and bearing that in mind, do you think your health is central to its business model? I don't think so.

Generally, the food industry's aim is making money, not focusing on your health. Always remember this when making choices about what you buy.

Let's have a look at 'low fat' products. I don't mean naturally low fat food (like an apple), I mean items like low fat yoghurt – there's a big difference.

Low fat products generally have added sugar and/ or refined white carbs. As a result, they release their glucose very quickly. This, in turn, leads to insulin being produced and fat being laid down. High blood glucose and insulin cause a rebound low blood sugar – this makes you very hungry and drives you to eat more.

But there are other things that these low fat products are doing to you to ramp up your appetite. Sugar can be addictive – driving some people to eat lots of refined carbs and sugar. Low fat products are often nutrient-deficient. You now know that this can cause you to be malnourished and increase your appetite. On top of all that are chemical 'additives' – these too can drive your appetite up.

Eating a lot of refined, low fat 'food' will drive you to eat more. This is great news for the food industry because they make more money out of you. But it's bad news for your waistline and health.

If your food needs a label there's a good chance it's not going to be good for you. But if you do eat this sort of food, check the label. The biggest ingredients are listed first; where does sugar appear?

Low fat is sold to us as a way to be healthy, to have good heart health and to lose weight. Even the medical profession have fallen for this somewhere along the line. We have been brainwashed by mass advertising to think that low fat products and low fat versions of real food help us.

Because so many people have fallen for it and buy so many of these processed low fat products, the food industry has a load of money to spend on advertising to brainwash us even more.

When fat is taken out of food, it has to be replaced by something else, otherwise there's not much left to eat!

Generally, a low fat diet leads to an increase in:
- Sugar and/or artificial chemical sweeteners
- Refined white carbs (e.g. white rice is lower in fat compared to its wholegrain counterpart and you have to eat more of it to feel full)

You know that refined carbs and sugar cause fat storage due to the necessary insulin response to control the high blood sugar they create.

Artificial chemical sweeteners, like aspartame, are definitely not your friend. They may be zero calories but they're chemicals that have been developed in a lab. Unnatural chemicals can do funny and strange things in your body, including causing weight gain! Yes, zero calorie and low sugar products can actually contribute to weight gain. These chemical sweeteners do this by stimulating your appetite, increasing carbohydrate cravings, and they stimulate fat storage.

The food industry spends a fortune on advertising its products. It can do this because it makes so much money from you buying their 'food'. It wants you to buy more so it can make even more profit. It wants you to get hooked on sugar (more coming on this) so you keep coming back for more, to keep lining their pockets. They don't care about you and your health. They don't care about your family's health; they have no concern for your children. If they did, they wouldn't target you and your family with disease-causing, fattening food.

When did you last see an apple being advertised? An apple is low fat. Why shouldn't it be advertised just like low fat crisps, cakes and biscuits? The simple answer is, there's no fortune to be made from apples. Who makes a pig out of themselves on apples? You just don't do it, do you? Therefore, you don't buy loads of apples and stuff yourself on them. But it's easy to go crazy and eat loads of refined and processed food, isn't it?

Imagine the advertising experts sitting down with the big food companies. They've come up with a new product. It's full of sugar and refined carbs, but because it's low fat they know most people will fall for it. They just need to decide on their target market. The target might be a child - your child. It might be the serial dieter who's been brainwashed into thinking low fat products are good for them. The target might be someone concerned with their heart, because they've had a heart attack.

The advertisers will literally be painting a *target* on your or your child's head. Then they will take aim with their advertising campaign to get you/your children hooked on food that will contribute to an early death. How does it make you feel to be hunted down like this by the food industry?

All in all, the low fat craze has been a fantastic opportunity for the food industry.

When you buy anything that's been made into a low fat product you're being manipulated for profit. The food industry and advertisers have hit their *target* every time you buy this sort of stuff. Keep the wool pulled back over your eyes and don't fall for this anymore.

The human body has no need whatsoever for refined carbs and sugar, but they're all over the place because the food industry loves them. It loves sugar for several reasons:
• It knows we like sweet things so it's an easy sell
• Sugar is a really cheap ingredient (more profit)
• Sugar extends the shelf life of products it appears in (more profit)

But most of all:
• Sugar is addictive

You could be addicted to sugar without realising it. If you are you'll keep coming back for more, and as you do that you spend more.

Many 'food products' made by the food industry are empty. They don't have real nutritional value – that value has been refined/removed. Empty foods make the people who eat them feel empty. It can be tempting for some people to fill this empty feeling with more food, which only continues the cycle.

You cannot rely on the food industry to give you accurate information about their products. It makes me laugh when I hear of calls to improve food labelling. If it needs a label it's probably not going to be good for you – end of story! When you choose to eat food that needs a label you take your chances!

It's up to you to educate yourself about the food you put in your body. That way, you can confidently safeguard your health, and your family's. You can stop being manipulated by advertising, stop being a *target*, and stop being compelled to eat food that's destroying your health.

There's only one winner when you eat unnatural, processed and refined food, and that isn't you. How does it feel knowing you're making the people who are deliberately *targeting* you and your children with health destroying food rich? They know what they're doing to you and they don't care. Now you know what they're doing, what are you going to do about it?

This isn't the end to the tricks they pull, I'm afraid there's more coming up later. But by the end of the book it will become clear how to make much better choices to safeguard your health.

18. Are You Addicted?

First some definitions:
- Addictive – (a drug or habit) causing addiction
- Addiction – the fact or process of being addicted
- Addicted – unable to do without a thing

I'm sure you will all recognise these things as potentially addictive:
- Alcohol
- Nicotine
- Hard drugs, like heroin

You may drink alcohol but not be addicted to it. Not everybody who uses an addictive substance becomes addicted. Most people who smoke are addicted, evident by the fact they can't stop.

But what about these things - do you recognise these as addictive substances?
- Sugar and white, refined carbs
- Conventional wheat
- Caffeine

These are all potentially addictive substances. But just because you use them doesn't mean you're addicted to them, but it might be worth giving it some thought as to whether you are addicted or not. After all, an addict has to recognise they have a problem before they can do anything about it.

I remember being sat in my GP surgery one day with a married couple. The wife had brought her husband in, to try and convince him to get help for his drink problem, which he clearly had. It was easy to see, looking from the outside. But he was in denial, reassuring me that although he drank a lot, he had it under control and could stop any time he wanted; he was just choosing not to. He couldn't see that he had a problem. Either that, or he wasn't ready to admit it to others yet. Maybe he hadn't even admitted it to himself.

The interesting thing about this consultation was when he turned the tables on his wife and suggested she get help with her addiction to food. According to him, she ate far too much and didn't know when to stop. She hotly denied she had a problem with food. However, she was very overweight and didn't like being that way.

I probably had two addicts in front of me. Neither were going to make any changes at that point in time because neither recognised they had a problem.

Keep your mind open at this point about yourself. It's only when you're open to possibilities that you stand a chance of seeing something that may have been hidden to you until now. You can keep this private, you don't need to share these thoughts with anyone.

Let's bring this back to food. Would you have a hissy fit if you were told you could never eat an apple or a banana ever again? Maybe you like apples and bananas and will be disappointed if one of them had to go, but I suspect you'd get by and survive. How about if it was bread, chocolate, caffeine or alcohol that had to go? Does that cause a different feeling?

When you eat or drink, are you satisfying a genuine hunger or thirst? Or are you relieving a discomfort of some kind?

What do I mean by that? I'm going to use a 'shoe' analogy to get my point across.

Ladies, have you ever been on a night out in shoes that look great but kill your feet? Gentlemen, have you ever squeezed yourself into trousers that are a bit tight and uncomfortable because they look good? How does it feel when you get home and can take the excruciating things off?

Would you put yourself through this discomfort if you were staying at home by yourself? I doubt it, because that would mean the only reason you wore the uncomfortable shoes or trousers was to enjoy the feeling of taking them off. That would be silly.

Do you regularly have strong cravings towards particular foods, such as bread, cereals, sweet things, snacks made of refined white carbs, chips, crisps, bagels, chocolate?

Is this a genuine hunger for food (because if it was, why would you be drawn to stuff like this time and time again?), or is something else going on?

No doubt when you satisfy your 'hunger' or craving by eating something like bread or something sweet like chocolate, you feel better. That's because you may have corrected a low blood sugar situation caused by the last lot you had, or had another fix in your addiction to sugar (remember all carbs are ultimately sugar). But this nice feeling is relatively short-lived as you're plunged back into low blood sugar again, and as your 'hit' wears off.

You've set yourself up nicely for your next craving of white, refined carbs and/or sugar. So, are you eating these 'foods' to satisfy genuine hunger, or are you relieving a discomfort (like taking off the shoes or trousers)?

If you eat a lot of wheat, refined white carbs, and/ or sugar, spend a bit of time thinking about this. As these are unnatural foods they have unnatural effects within your body. If you think you may have a problem, it's not your fault. Your body has simply succumbed to an addictive substance, but unlike heroin, you didn't know it was addictive so didn't see the danger.

You have to see your problem first before you can do anything about it. The doing something about it involves the gradual change onto real, whole foods as mentioned before. It also involves being conscious to what's going on inside you and thinking about what could have caused you to feel the way you do. Question your cravings. What could be driving them? This is all stuff to ponder in your notebook.

Refined sugar, refined carbs, and conventional wheat:
- Are abnormal foods
- Are bad for your health and can make you ill
- Can be addictive
- Make you fat

Caffeine

You may wonder why I'm including a section about caffeine in a book that's predominantly about fat loss. The penny will drop by the end of this short section.

If you drink caffeine, either as tea, coffee, or in soft drinks, why do you have it? These are some of the reasons people have given me:
- *I like it*
- *It's a thirst quencher*
- *It gives me energy*
- *It makes me mentally sharper*

- *It helps me to get going in the morning*
- *It's a sociable thing to do with friends*
- *It's a habit*

Before you read any further have a look at the following sleep chart.

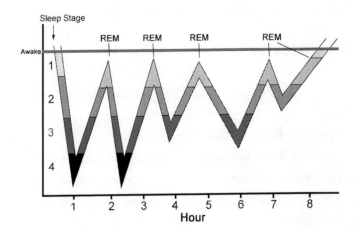

As you can see, you have various stages of sleep. In addition to REM sleep (which is when you dream) you have varying levels regarding the depth of your sleep. Stage two is deeper than stage one, stage three is deeper than two. Stage four is deepest of all, and you have about two episodes of this during a night's sleep.

Stage four is really important, because that's when a lot of rest and recuperation takes place. Without this, you'll feel sluggish and tired the next day.

Everyone knows that drinking caffeine close to

bedtime can stop you sleeping. But did you know that regular caffeine intake can prevent you getting any stage four sleep? It's possible to be asleep all night and not get any stage four sleep, leaving you feeling unrefreshed and tired. Even if you drink a lot of caffeine and can get to sleep easily you may be still wrecking your sleep without realising it.

The Caffeine Cycle

- Your sleep is poor because you drink caffeine regularly
- You feel tired in the morning as a result
- You drink some caffeine in the morning to try and get yourself going (this might be a habit by now)
- The effect is short-lived because you're sleep deprived
- You drink more caffeine as the day goes on to keep going (or just out of habit because you no longer give it any conscious thought)
- It's impossible to sleep well because you're not getting any stage four sleep
- You feel lethargic and sluggish in the morning...

Feeling tired every day isn't going to help you make better choices regarding your food, and it certainly isn't going to make you feel like doing any exercise – this is why I've included caffeine in this book.

Do you think the caffeine industry is aware of

this? Of course they are! The more people that are
unknowingly addicted to caffeine the more money they
make. How much money is spent on advertising tea,
coffee and soft drinks? Have you got another target on
your head?

Caffeine Does Not Give You Energy

It's a common misconception that caffeine gives
you energy. It doesn't. What it does is stimulate
your adrenal glands, causing them to release
stress hormones, including adrenalin. These stress
hormones then trigger a release of glucose from your
glycogen stores – this is why you feel a bit of a lift
after caffeine. In effect, caffeine 'borrows' energy from
your adrenal glands.

Going back to when humans were hunter-gatherers,
there were occasions when they needed an instant
energy rush - for example, if they were being hunted
for dinner. In this situation they would feel stressed,
and as a result, their adrenal glands would release
adrenalin. This would then cause a glucose rush and
give instant energy to run away.

Caffeine has the same effect. Regular caffeine use
means repeated stimulation of your adrenals. If you
keep doing this, at some point, your adrenals won't
have anything left. The result is that you feel tired all
the time.

So, caffeine wrecks your sleep, and over time, your adrenals too. This can mean you feel fatigued a lot. Obviously, the more caffeine you drink, the more you risk this.

Lack of energy means:
- You're less likely to make changes
- You're less likely to exercise
- You're less likely to succeed

If you drink more than a couple of cups of caffeine every day AND you feel your energy isn't what it should be, consider that caffeine could be the cause.

The other thing to consider with caffeine is that it dehydrates you, because it's a diuretic. This means you produce a greater volume of urine compared to the volume of fluid you drank in the cup of tea or coffee. Remember: your fat-busting enzymes need you well hydrated to do their work efficiently. Caffeine doesn't help here, it hinders.

Cutting Down
If you drink a lot of caffeine don't cut down or stop abruptly. You could make yourself quite ill. Here's a comment from one of my blog readers:

'I've got a caffeine horror story... a few years ago I used to go and stay with my sister and her family in her house in Blackpool. The funny thing was, every

single time I used to go and stay with her, after a couple of days, I'd start to get a headache, which would get worse and worse. I'd eventually become really sick and end up vomiting. My mum and stepdad used to experience exactly the same thing when they visited and we were at a total loss as to why going to stay with my sister made us all so ill.

A couple of years later she moved to a different house, and we noticed that when we went to stay we no longer became ill. We assumed it must have been something to do with the old house, until I went shopping with her during a visit. As she put a jar of coffee into her trolley she remarked that when they lived at their old house she always used to buy decaffeinated coffee, but since they'd moved she hadn't bothered and now bought ordinary coffee.

The penny dropped straight away. Every time we'd visited her at her old house we were all withdrawing from caffeine! My mum and stepdad drink loads of coffee and so do I. It's scary, really - and time I addressed this addiction.'

Cutting down gradually is the way to go. I would suggest cutting one cup out every week or two – do it slowly, there's no need to rush.

It's worth trying, at least. So many people on my course have been amazed at how much more energy they had when they cut caffeine considerably (and hydrated themselves properly).

Alcohol

I'm not going to spend a lot of time here, otherwise I'll risk going off track. There's so much I could say about alcohol.

In a nutshell, alcohol is packed with empty calories. By that, I mean it provides a lot of calories but very little in the way of the other ingredients needed to burn those calories. It has practically no nutritional value. It's so easy to consume a large amount of calories because alcohol doesn't fill you up. I find that many people completely underestimate how much they're drinking, and therefore how many calories they take in.

Bearing in mind that alcohol is an addictive substance, and that 90% of people in western countries drink it, there's probably a lot of hidden addiction out there. How would you feel if you couldn't have a drink for two months? If this is genuinely no problem and you could easily start right now, that's great (why don't you do it?); you haven't got a problem. But if you feel uncomfortable about that prospect for any reason, ask yourself why. We all know alcohol is addictive. It's just something for you to think about.

I see many people during my GP work who have a problem with alcohol. Some of them know they're not fully in control, some of them say they need it to help with stress. Most of them don't fit the stereotype of an alcoholic. Some of them don't drink every day, but they can't easily go a week without a drink.

Our guidelines in the UK for safe alcohol consumption are 14 units a week for women and 21 units for men. It's advised to have no more than 3 units in one sitting for women and 4 for men. It is also recommended to spread your intake over the week, and have at least two days off. This gives your body the recovery time it needs.

Drinking above these levels on a regular basis means you will be causing your body some sort of damage, but it will probably be a few years before you find out what that is. Alcohol ages you. You can see this in your skin, but it's also going on inside too. Alcohol contributes to heart disease and cancer.

In addition to the empty calories, alcohol hampers your fat loss effort for two other reasons. It causes low blood sugar and this increases your appetite, so you eat more. So, not only have you taken in a load of calories with the alcohol itself, it's going to drive you to eat more than you need. Also, it strips nutrients from your body. Alcohol is toxic, and your body has to work hard to break it down and clear it from your system. A lot of nutrients are used during this process.

If you don't feel fully in control of your drinking consider getting a copy of this great book: The Easy Way to Control Alcohol, by Allen Carr.

I think the UK guidelines for safe alcohol use are pretty sensible. I see no need to stop drinking alcohol, unless you want to. If you're drinking according to the guidelines, this fits a healthy lifestyle and doesn't impact on you achieving your ideal weight.

19. Fat – The Good, The Bad And The Ugly

Although I'm focusing on fat in this chapter, I'll revisit it in the next, when I move on to protein.

Fats Are Vital To Health

During our evolution as humans it was a diet high in fat that was responsible for the massive development of our brains. This suggests that fat is really important. In fact, good quality fat in your diet is vital for a healthy brain and nervous system.

Fat is used to make every single cell in your body. Fat is needed for building, rebuilding and maintaining your cell membranes. Cell membranes have to keep the watery stuff inside the cell and the watery stuff outside the cell separate. Only fat can do this. Fat is used for many other vital things too, like making hormones and neurotransmitters in your brain.

Bearing this in mind, low fat diets are crazy. Human beings cannot be healthy without eating a decent amount of *quality* fat in their diet. Deficiencies in quality fat lead to all sorts of illnesses, and even obesity.

Fat Keeps Hunger At Bay For Longer

Hunger is influenced by the types of food you eat. Even though fat contains twice as many calories as carbs it keeps your hunger satisfied three times longer.

Here is how long the various food groups can keep your hunger at bay:
- High fat meal – 5-8 hours
- High protein meal – 3-5 hours
- Complex carb meal – 2-3 hours
- Refined carb/sugar meal – can be as little as 30 minutes

This is yet another reason why the low fat message is barking mad. But, like carbs, fats aren't equal either. The key is to make sure you eat good quality fat that helps your health, not the types of fat harmful to your health. The low fat message tends to lump all fat together, but they're not the same.

The Good

In fact, these aren't just good, they're really good. These are your essential fatty acids. They're called essential because, without them, you can't enjoy good health; in fact, problems will be around the corner if you're without them for a significant length of time.

Things linked to a deficiency, or imbalance, of essential fatty acids include dry skin, hair loss, being prone to infections, arthritis, cancer, heart disease, low metabolic rate and obesity. Yes, a deficiency in fat can help make you fat!

Getting good fats into your body regularly gives you soft skin that doesn't need moisturising. It makes your hair shine. It supports a healthy immune system that helps protect you from infections and cancers. They help keep your joints moving smoothly and pain free. And they keep your metabolism ticking over nicely, helping you lose your body fat and keep it off.

The essential fatty acids are omega 6 and the omega 3s. They're found in fresh and unrefined whole goods and also good quality meat and fish.

It's highly unusual to be deficient of omega 6. Due to changes in our food you're likely to have too much of this, in relation to omega 3s. The reason for this will become evident in the next chapter, which is about protein.

It's very common for people in western countries to be deficient of the omega 3s, due to how our diet has changed. So, this is what I'll concentrate on.

The omega 3s are:
- ALA – alpha-Linolenic acid
- DHA – Docoshexaenoic acid
- EPA – Eicosapentaenoic acid

ALA is the plant form of omega 3 and your body converts this to DHA and EPA; in these forms it becomes useful to your body's needs. ALA is found in:
- Flaxseed (linseed) – high amounts
- Hemp seed
- Chia seed
- Walnuts
- Dark green, leafy vegetables

If you eat a vegetarian diet, and especially if you eat a vegan diet, include these things in what you eat on a regular basis.

DHA and EPA are found in meat and oily fish that have been fed a diet that's natural to them.

These really good fats go off quite quickly, so they

have to be eaten when fresh. They're also destroyed by temperatures significantly above boiling and they're broken down quickly by exposure to light and air. For these reasons, you won't find any essential fats in processed, refined and packaged food. They're deliberately removed because they go off quickly, making the food rancid. That's no good for the shelf life of processed food.

You find the essential fats EPA and DHA in real, fresh foods, and really good sources are:
- Quality meats – see the next chapter
- Wild, oily fish, like salmon, mackerel, sardines and tuna
- Good quality eggs – see next chapter

Saturated fats have a foot in two camps, depending on their source. Saturated fats found in butter and meats tend to burn really well as fuel, because they're relatively small molecules. They're known as 'short chain' fatty acids. Unless they're eaten in complete excess, saturated fats DO NOT MAKE YOU FAT! Neither do they cause heart disease. Here's an extract from a blog I wrote in October 2013:

British Medical Journal Article about Saturated Fat and Heart Disease

Dr Malhotra's article in the BMJ – 'Saturated Fat is Not the Issue' highlights something important.

Scientists know that abnormal fats (like trans-fats) that are found in margarines, fried, fast and processed foods, lead to heart disease. Margarine is losing so far in the margarine vs. butter debate.

When we doctors look at your cholesterol result we look at a number of things; here are two of them:
1. *HDL = 'good cholesterol'*
2. *LDL = 'bad cholesterol'*

It is widely believed that saturated fat (the fat found in butter, dairy products and meat) increases LDL, i.e. 'bad' cholesterol. It does indeed increase LDL.

However, what this blood test result doesn't tell us is that there is more than one type of LDL. Dr Malhotra mentions two of them:
1. *type A LDL – these levels are linked to saturated fat*
2. *type B LDL – these are linked to carbohydrate and sugar intake*

Here's the interesting thing – it is type B that's linked to heart disease, not type A...

This means that saturated fat isn't particularly linked to heart disease, but the wrong sort of carbohydrates is. Just as we already know that abnormal fats, like those found in margarine, are too.

Before agriculture humans ate a high fat and low carb

diet. Much of the fat was saturated fat. Given the fact that humans made it through such as ice ages and got to where we are today, saturated fat can't be the evil thing it's made out to be. And scientific study is proving that.

One of the keys to enjoying fat in your diet is not to eat them with significant amounts of carbs at the same time. In nature, fat always comes with protein – not carbs. Fat naturally comes along with protein in meat, fish, eggs, seeds and nuts. When eaten in this natural way it won't make you fat.

The Bad

When you eat too many carbs for your current energy needs and glycogen stores to cope with, the rest are converted to fat for storage. They are converted to saturated fat. This type of saturated fat is not the same as the saturated fat you eat.

When carbs are converted to saturated fat they become 'long chain' fatty acids. The saturated fat you eat in meat and dairy is 'short chain'. There's a big difference. Long chain fatty acids are more difficult to burn as energy, so are more prone to be left in storage if there are easier things to burn up. There will nearly always be easier energy to burn, like the energy from the meal or drink you've just had.

This kind of saturated fat is linked to heart disease and makes you fat. But it doesn't come from fat in your diet, it comes from carbs. Hunter-gatherers don't have this sort of saturated fat in their bodies, because they eat very little carbs.

The mix of carbs and fat - found in cakes, biscuits, doughnuts, ice cream, pastries - is completely unnatural to your human physiology. The carb and fat mix is a man-made product that doesn't exist in nature. In nature, fat comes with protein, not carbs.

This mix is completely abnormal to the human physiology. You don't feel full when eating this kind of stuff, so your body doesn't know when to stop. This is why you can keep eating and eating this kind of stuff and not feel full. Take Pringles for example: 'Once you pop, you just can't stop!' Do you think the food industry knows this happens when you eat this sort of 'food'?

Another experiment done on the poor rat caught my interest. The first group was fed on sugar foods only. The second group was fed on fat only. Both of these groups appeared to stop eating when satisfied. This was assumed because food was available for them all day, but after eating a meal-sized portion they would stop eating, even though food was freely available. They would go back for more later, presumably when they were hungry again. They maintained a normal body weight.

The third group was fed a diet of 50/50 fat and sugar. You don't find this combination in nature, it doesn't exist. Like us, the rat isn't equipped to deal with it and this resulted in this group grazing all day. They didn't appear to know when to stop and got really fat.

Obviously I'm not saying it's okay to eat a diet that's 100% based on sugar or 100% based on fat. Either of these diets would cause severe deficiencies in the essential nutrients in a short space of time, and you would get ill. But I think this experiment demonstrates the problem of the man-made combination of fat and carbs when it comes to weight gain.

When you eat fat with what it naturally comes with – meat, fish, eggs, cheese, nuts and seeds - you get full and know when to stop. When you eat fat packaged up with carbs in a man-made product – cakes, pastries, biscuits, doughnuts - your body doesn't know where the off switch is, because these foods are alien to your physiology. You can easily, and seriously, overdo your calorie intake without even feeling full.

The Very Ugly

The down-right awful for your health fats are the

man-made hydrogenated and trans-fats. These are not found in natural foods; humans have not evolved to cope with them, that's why they cause so many problems to health.

Hydrogenation is the process that makes vegetable oils solid at room temperature. Think about it: something drastic has to happen to the structure of the fat to make oil, which is liquid, into something solid. The result is something highly unnatural. This is what happens to make margarine. During the process of hydrogenation, some trans-fats are formed too. Trans-fats are also formed when ANY vegetable oil is fried. Eating these abnormal man-made fats is not good for you and contributes to fat gain.

Where did margarine come from? Emperor Napoleon the Third of France had a lot to do with it. He offered a prize to anyone who could find a satisfactory alternative to butter that would be suitable for the armed forces and the lower classes. It had to be cheap and not go off. In 1813 a French chemist made margarine in his lab.

It wasn't until World War Two that margarine became popular, due to shortages of butter. Butter, as you know, is yellow. Margarine is actually white; it has to be dyed to be accepted and palatable, even to this day. After World War Two, advertising took off and there were big attempts to make it taste like butter.

Now many people have margarine in their fridges, thinking they're making a better choice for their health. This is the power of advertising at work. Many people have been brainwashed into thinking margarine is healthier than butter. How can something that was invented in a lab possibly be healthier than something natural like butter? Your body knows what to do with the saturated fat in butter. Humans evolved eating saturated fat. It's natural to your diet. It does not know what to do with hydrogenated fat in margarine. This is alien and unnatural.

Hydrogenated vegetable fats are found in a lot of processed food. They'll be found in pastries, cakes, biscuits, snacks. Check the labels of the processed food you have and see if they're there.

Trans-fats are found in all fried food, if the oil used to fry was vegetable oil. This is because the structure of vegetable oil changes under high temperatures. Trans-fats are completely abnormal in natural food. The human body can't cope well with many of these.

Like hydrogenated fats, trans-fats don't go off. This is marvellous news to the food industry. Processed food with trans-fats and hydrogenated fats takes ages and ages to go off, so it has a long shelf life. Good news for the food industry's profits. You often find these abnormal fats combined with refined carbs and sugar.

It's a recipe for bad health and weight problems.

Your ability to deal with these abnormal fats is limited. You can cope with a small, infrequent amount fine, but when your intake exceeds your ability to deal with them, two things will happen:

- They will be put into storage – you put weight on
- They will be used to build your cells – you could get ill

When your body has better fats to use to build things like cells and hormones, these abnormal fats will be sent for storage. Your body would prefer not to have this problem, so if it can ignore it, it will. It can just sit in storage.

If you haven't been eating a good supply of *quality* fats your body will attempt to use these abnormal fats for vital structures and functions. They're not normal, natural fats and so are not designed for this, which is why you can get ill when you eat this kind of stuff regularly. If you try to build a house with bricks that don't fit together, it's not going to last like one that's built with proper, natural-shaped bricks, is it?

Cast your mind back to what happens when carbohydrates are refined. The vast majority of vegetable oils on the supermarket shelf have been refined and processed. This means the essential fatty acids have gone (because they go off and reduce the shelf life) and most of the essential nutrients have gone too.

Virgin (and extra virgin) olive oil is the only mass produced oil that has not been refined. This means it's the only mass produced oil that's healthy to eat. A word of caution though - if you fry with it, you'll create a load of trans-fats and it will no longer be healthy. When you fry, use butter. Saturated fats are stable at high temperatures and therefore do not turn into the harmful trans-fats.

When it comes to your excess body fat and health, the fats that work against you are the ones that aren't naturally found in nature. It's not necessarily the case to never eat these, but you'll do your health a big favour by keeping them to a minimum. As a general guide to avoiding them:

• Use butter instead of margarine
• Fry with butter (or coconut oil, which is a saturated fat) and not vegetable oil
• Generally keep fried foods to a minimum
• Foods that are a mix of carbs and fats (cakes, biscuits, pastries) are likely to have hydrogenated fat in them – another reason to keep them to a minimum

But when you eat healthily most of the time, your body can cope with the odd indulgence, so don't feel like these are on a forbidden list.

Fats in Summary

Fat has got a bad name, and this isn't fair. Some fats are very bad for us, but it seems all have been tarnished with the same brush.

It makes sense to avoid, or keep to a minimum, the abnormal, man-made, hydrogenated fats. You will also do your body a service by keeping to a minimum the carb and fat mix found in things like cakes, puddings and crisps. These two things often go hand in hand and are found in the foods most people already know aren't ideal for health and a svelte waistline.

The important message in this chapter is not to be frightened of eating, and enjoying, healthy fats. Your body needs them to be healthy. Your metabolism needs them to run smoothly and actually burn your body fat.

You'll learn more detail in the next chapter about healthy fat choices. But eating fat where it is found naturally in nature is the general guide to follow. For example, the majority of calories in avocados are from fat, but this is a very healthy thing to eat. I eat one most days. Low fat salad dressings are nonsensical – make your own, with plenty of healthy extra virgin olive oil (you'll find a recipe at the back of the book).

In the next chapter I'll cover more about how to get

good sources of fat, packaged up as Mother Nature intended it to be eaten – with protein.

20. Protein

Protein builds, maintains and replaces the tissues in your body. Your muscles, internal organs and skin are largely made up of protein. When you digest protein, it's broken down into its building blocks: amino acids. Your body uses these amino acids to make the various specialised proteins you need in your body. Muscle protein is different to skin protein because different sequences and different amino acids are used.

There are about twenty amino acids, and your body can make most of them. But it can't make eight of them. These are known as the essential amino acids. You have to get these from your diet. This is important to bear in mind if you eat a vegetarian or vegan diet.

You get 'complete' protein from animal and fish sources. Complete means that it contains all the essential amino acids. You get 'incomplete' protein from plant sources. You can get complete proteins from plant sources by combining them well, e.g. beans and wholegrain rice give all your essential amino acids in one meal (such as in a vegetarian chilli).

Essential Fats Revisited

Your essential fats are omega 6 and omega 3. For best health, these should be eaten in a ratio of 1:1. This means, for every one omega 6 fatty acid you eat, you should have one omega 3 fatty acid to balance it.

Many people in western countries are deficient in omega 3. This can happen for two reasons, or, usually, a combination of the two. You might not be eating enough of omega 3 in the first place. However, if you have too much omega 6, compared with omega 3, the ratio is all wrong and this can make you deficient too. Things have to be in their correct quantities to work - for example, if you're making bread and use four times the amount of water you need...it's not going to work, is it? In effect, your excess water has made you deficient of flour.

Remember – a deficiency of omega 3 can contribute to weight gain. Getting the correct ratio of essential fats is relevant to common protein sources today.

The Problem With Most Meat And Some Fish

It's difficult to always know how fresh meat and fish is. Sometimes, meat has been stored in a frozen state for a long time. The longer it's stored the more essential nutrients are lost, especially the good fats. Knowing exactly where your food has come from helps with this. Having a good butcher and fishmonger on hand is ideal. The quality of meat, fish, eggs, and dairy depends on what the creatures were fed on.

Many farmed animals are not fed their natural diet, so how can they be healthy? Animals are routinely fed abnormal food to make them grow more quickly and to fatten them up. For example, cows aren't supposed to eat grains, they're supposed to eat only grass. It's interesting that farm animals are fed grains to fatten them up, yet we're encouraged to eat them to lose weight.

This is the same with fish: farmed salmon and sea bass are fed things abnormal to their usual diet.

The problem with animals and fish that haven't eaten what they were meant to eat is that the fats in their bodies aren't what they're supposed to be. In a naturally fed cow (exclusively grass fed), the ratio of omega 3 to 6 is as it should be, 1:1. A cow that has been fed a 'junk food' diet with a lot of grain to fatten it up can have a ratio of omega 3 to 6 as high as 1:40!

The balance of essential fatty acids is all wrong; it's like having too much water compared with flour when you're making bread. When you've got too much omega 6 it makes you deficient of omega 3.

One result of omega 3 deficiency is weight gain. So

your choices of protein are important for both your health and your weight.

Better Protein Choices Have Healthier Fat Content

Red meat has a bad name when it comes to general health. This isn't because red meat is inherently bad, it's because the way it's farmed has turned it into something unhealthy. Animals fed on a diet to fatten them end up with too much omega 6 inside them, compared to omega 3. This has a knock-on effect to the people who eat this on a regular basis.

The best red meat you can eat is organic and exclusively grass fed. This meat has the correct balance of fats because the animal has been fed properly. You can order this online if you can't buy it locally, but good butchers do sell this.

Meats to keep to an absolute minimum are processed meats – like bacon. This isn't a normal or natural way to eat meat and there are links to cancer in people who eat this kind of meat a lot, particularly bowel cancer.

For similar reasons, free range organic chickens are much better for you. They've eaten a diet very close to what's normal for them. Free range chickens tend to be smaller. This is because they're made up of more muscle and little fat. Most chickens on the supermarket shelf are obese, bloated birds. They've been fed an abnormal diet of corn to fatten them up as quickly as possible, and haven't been able to exercise. This results in a completely wrong balance of fats within their bodies.

Wild fish is good for you. Farmed fish isn't particularly good for you. Farmed fish are not fed on a diet that's healthy or normal. Again, they're fed on things to get them to grow and fatten up as quickly as possible, and as a result, the balance of fats is all wrong.

In the UK we eat a lot of farmed salmon, having been tricked into thinking this is a healthy option. Have you even seen wild salmon and farmed salmon next to each other at your supermarket or fishmongers? If you haven't seen the difference before have a look the next time you get the opportunity.

Wild Atlantic salmon is almost red. It's a very deep orange. Its farmed counterpart is a pasty shade of orange by comparison. The difference is largely due to the increased fat content and decreased protein in the farmed fish. Farmed fish is very fatty, but has an abnormal balance of fats, i.e. too much omega 6 and too little omega 3.

Yet again the food industry is up to its tricks. Salmon is promoted as a great source of omega 3. This is true if the salmon is wild, but not true if it's farmed.

Eggs

Eggs can be a great source of complete protein and fat soluble vitamins, providing they're quality eggs. What makes a quality egg? A good quality egg comes from a good quality chicken. A good quality chicken is one that has a diet normal to a chicken, and which can exercise.

Left pretty much to its own devices, a chicken will forage for its own food (outside), eating insects that it finds within the grass and on the ground. A chicken like this will lay fabulous quality eggs that have a deep orange yolk. These eggs have a great balance of fats in them and are also a good source of protein.

The more yellow the yolk the more grain (usually corn) the chicken has been fed (an abnormal diet for a chicken). The more insipid the colour of the yolk, the less nutritious the egg will be for you, regardless of whether it's organic or not. Eggs don't need to be organic; you don't get 'organic insects'. The best eggs come from truly free range chickens – those that can feed themselves outside on insects.

So, the darker the yolk, the better quality the egg. Most commercial chickens will be fed on some grain too, so for that reason, organic are better. I'm lucky that I know several people who have their own chickens that get to wander about and feed themselves. I buy these eggs whenever I can. When I have to resort to shop-bought, I go for organic and free range. From experience, I know these ones are likely to have a more orange yolk. I get them from local grocers who get their eggs from a local farm.

Dairy

I find milk a funny one. Humans are the only species to drink milk in adulthood. In addition to that, we drink a different species' milk. Cow's milk is meant for baby cows, not adult humans.

There are a multitude of health problems related to cow's milk consumption, including allergies, digestive problems and excessive mucus production. It's beyond the scope of this book, so I'll limit this to general principles.

Milk has been messed around with and processed, and as a result, isn't as good for you as it could be. Fat soluble vitamins are found only in fat. When you take the fat out of milk you also take out these nutrients too. The fat is taken out because you've been sold an untruth, that saturated fat is bad for you and makes you fat. You now know that the saturated fat in your diet isn't a problem, so these low fat and processed versions are unnecessary. You're basically choosing a nutritionally-deficient version when you choose low fat options of milk, yoghurt and cheese.

Eat the full fat versions (and get more nutrition) - in moderation - and enjoy them.

What the cow eats is reflected in the milk it produces. For this reason, organic is better, because you're not going to get all the pesticides and similar rubbish you get in 'normal' milk.

Vegetable Sources Of Protein

Protein seems to be synonymous with meat but you don't have to eat animal and fish sources of protein to get your full quota - but you do need to make sure you get enough. This is pretty easy to do, provided you take some care over it.

Even if you eat meat and fish regularly, the vegetable sources of protein are really good things to include in your diet, to give you variety.

Nuts are a brilliant source of both protein and good fats. You get most benefit if you eat them raw; this is because the fat within them retains its great health qualities. Raw nuts make a great snack between meals if you get peckish. There are plenty of different sorts: peanuts, cashew nuts, Brazil nuts, walnuts, macadamia nuts.

Although you get the best health benefits from eating them raw, you can still get plenty of protein benefit when they're cooked; for example, in nut butters.

Seeds are another fantastic source of protein and great fats. Again, you get full benefit eating them in their raw state. You can mix a few sunflower seeds or pumpkin seeds in with some nuts to make a very healthy snack.

If you fancy making your own bread, you could increase the protein content by adding your favourite nuts and seeds. Because a crust forms around the bread when it's cooking, the inside cooks more by being steamed. This means the temperature inside doesn't tend to get high enough to ruin the great fats inside the seeds and nuts. So, a spelt or rye loaf could end up being a great source of protein with these included.

Other great sources of proteins are peas, beans and lentils. When these are eaten with grains, like rice, you get your full complement of protein. A veggie chilli, based on beans and served with wholegrain rice, or a lentil curry served with wholegrain rice, makes a meal with good protein content. Soups made out of split peas, hummus made out of chickpeas, and sesame seed paste are great too.

Whole grains are another good source of protein. You can use wholegrain spelt and rye. There is also wholegrain rice, barley and buckwheat. Quinoa is a particularly good source of protein.

You don't need animal based food to get more than enough protein in your diet, but it's a good idea to eat a good variety of the above foods to make sure you get all your essential amino acids.

Summary

Mother Nature provides you with many sources of protein to keep you fit and healthy. As you can see, protein comes with fat, so it's hard to consider one without the other. It's unusual for people in western countries to be short on protein, but due to modern farming methods, the fat that comes with the protein may have been completely changed. Many people end up being deficient of omega 3s.

Knowledge is the key when it comes to your health (actually, applying that knowledge is the real key).

You are now armed with the information you need to make better choices. You can't be fooled any more.

In the next section you'll learn about exercise. Don't worry, I'll break you in gently. Following that, I'll be tying together all the nutrition and exercise information, by explaining how the combination of the two gets your metabolism in top shape.

Part 4 – Exercise
21. Introduction

Humans living in the west aren't really designed for the world we live in. In the last few hundred years our world has changed dramatically, and over the last one hundred years almost everything about the way we live is different.

As a result of these changes, people are at their all-time heaviest, and as a consequence, disease levels are at epidemic proportions. This is only going to get worse in the coming decades, if people don't change.

Our ancestors evolved in the world they lived in. You have the same genes as your ancestors. Every day they had physical challenges that, along with the correct diet, kept their bodies lean, trim and muscular. Your hunter-gatherer ancestors didn't exercise as such, but they did a wide range of activities. To thrive and be healthy your body needs to do the same.

There are a few populations of hunter-gatherers in existence even now, giving researchers the opportunity to study them. The Hadza of north-central Tanzania are likely to be living very much like your ancestors did. There are about a thousand of them and 300-400 of them live as hunter-gatherers, much as their ancestors did tens of thousands of years ago.

They are the last full-time hunter-gatherers in Africa.

The Hadza tend to be lean. A man in his thirties will have a body fat percentage of 13%, and a woman, about 21%. Compare that to the average in the UK of 20% for a man and 32% for a woman. These figures are even higher in the US.

The Hadza do a mixture of activities. They walk quite a lot, they have regular short episodes of intense activity, e.g. when hunting, and they do activities that involve strength, e.g. climbing and chopping wood. This activity is interspersed with periods of relative inactivity, e.g. if they've been very active one day this may be followed by a day of rest.

This suggests that you need to be active to be healthy and slim, but there is room for the odd lazy day too (phew!).

There are some people who do a lot of exercise, but remain overweight. If you fall into this group you will just need to make a few tweaks if you want to trim down – to your diet, and maybe to the way you exercise too.

However, exercising overweight people are far healthier compared to their equally overweight couch potato counterparts. Even if you're still overweight you will fare a lot better with your health if you exercise.

One reason is because you'll have a larger muscle mass that tips the scales in the right direction, with regards to your metabolism (more coming up about that in the next chapter).

You might have your focus mainly on weight loss, but the benefits of exercise are far more reaching that just that. People who keep active and do some exercise regularly are less likely to get cancer than regularly sedentary people. One reason thought to be the case is that cancer does best and thrives in oxygen-poor states. An exercised body is in an oxygen-rich state.

When someone keeps active and exercises they bring lots of oxygen into their bodies with the deep breathing that exercise requires. Muscle contractions pump this oxygen-rich blood around your body. This is not a good environment for cancer, which is one reason you're less likely to succumb if you keep active.

But if you are someone who is exercising with the aim of fat loss, and not getting anywhere with this, how frustrating! What's going on here? It might be the way you are exercising, because not all exercise is equal. The key to exercising for fat loss is the *quality* of it over the *quantity*. But obviously you need to be looking at what you're eating too, because you can't exercise your way out of a bad diet.

22. Being Generally More Active

Hunter-gatherers are generally more active than the average western person, even though they have no formal exercise programme. The foundation of this activity is walking.

Going back to the Hadza: on average, they walk between four to seven miles per day (about 10,000 steps). Sometimes, they might do a big walk all in one go - for example, if they're hunting. Other times, it's made up of lots of short journeys. Other days they might do very little.

A number of studies (A meta-analysis of pedometer-based walking interventions and weight loss; Richardson CR1, Newton TL, Abraham JJ, Sen A, Jimbo M, Swartz AM; 2008 Jan-Feb) have been to carried out to investigate the effect of increased activity by walking (measured with a pedometer), without any changes to diet. These studies consistently show modest weight loss with regular increased walking.

One study wasn't looking specifically at weight loss. The researchers were more interested in the effect of increased walking on future heart disease.

One group was given a pedometer and required to walk an extra two thousand steps above and beyond what they would normally do. This could be done as a twenty minute walk, so not a great impact on their day. It could also be done as two or more shorter ones, reflecting simple things like parking your car further away from the shop's front door.

As the study went on, it was shown that the rate of heart disease in this group did fall. However, so did their weight by a modest amount. So, on a daily basis, a twenty minute walk caused these people to lose weight; they made no other changes. How easy would it be for you to have a short walk every day? This would be in addition to what you already do. You wouldn't even have to go out for a walk. There are ample opportunities every day to be a little more active.

There's a supermarket I sometimes go to. You have to go up a level to get into the shop. There are normal stairs and on either side of these there are escalators – one going up and one coming down. It never ceases to amaze me how many able-bodied people without trolleys are going up and down on these.

It comes down to what you do most of the time. I'm quite active and I would estimate that 95% of the time if I see where the stairs are (often they're hidden) I use them, rather than the escalators or lift. Sometimes I feel tired, lazy and just can't be bothered, so I choose the easy option. But it's what you do most of the time that counts.

By consistently choosing the stairs you can increase your average daily step rate.

When you go shopping, or to the gym or cinema – do you drive around for a few minutes to find the closest parking spot or do you drive to where you can see a few available spaces a fair distance away? I was meeting a friend to see a film and we pulled into the car park at the same time. I headed off to where I could see some spaces that were towards the back of the car park. We met at the door at the same time, even though parked much closer than I did (but she'd spent a while driving around looking for it). I obviously took more steps than my friend on this occasion.

By consistently not parking as close as possible (and wasting time doing so) to where you want to go, you increase your daily step rate.

How else could you walk more? Do you regularly make journeys that are less than a mile in your car rather than walking? If so, why? What's stopping you from walking?

23. Forget About 'Fat Burning Cardio'

When people want to lose weight many start some sort of exercise, like jogging or going to the gym.

Something that GPs have been 'prescribing' in recent years is exercise. In the area where I work this involves getting a discounted membership to a gym and initial help from an instructor. When I ask my patients what they're doing at the gym it usually involves 'cardio' work. This means exercising for a period of time while in the 'fat burning zone'. Essentially, this means keeping your heart rate between 60-70% of its maximum rate and exercising for at least 30 minutes, ideally more. (I feel bored just contemplating doing this!)

They might be walking or jogging on a treadmill for half an hour, or longer. Alternatively, they could be on an exercise bike, cross trainer or rowing machine. Some people prefer swimming.

Many people put in a tremendous amount of effort, exercising four-five times per week, but they remain overweight. This is hugely frustrating. Often, one of the reasons is that their diet hasn't changed; they're still eating the wrong sort of foods.

At the end of the day - *you can't exercise yourself out of a bad diet.*

However, if you're going to spend time and effort exercising you first need to know why you're doing it. If you're doing something for enjoyment, that's great, but if you're doing exercise with the aim of weight loss and/or health gain – then you want know your time and effort is well spent.

Exercising For Health

'Cardio' exercise, like jogging, long distance running or cycling, increases the endurance of your heart and lungs. This might sound good, but humans aren't designed for this. Hunter-gatherers didn't, and still don't, use their bodies in this way. They do a lot of walking but they don't go for a jog. Instead, they do short bursts of high intensity activity, like sprinting after, or away from, an animal. This challenges their heart and lungs to their maximum, not just 60-70%.

As you age, the cells in your lungs die off faster than you replace them, unless you're regularly challenging them. Your lungs are a bit like your muscles: if you don't use them, they get smaller and lose capacity. It is very much 'use it or lose it'. Your lungs also shrink as you get older, unless you're regularly doing something to keep them in shape.

As your lungs gradually shrink over the years, your stamina, strength and ability to fight off disease all reduce. In fact, the smaller your lungs get, the more at risk of death you are, of any cause.

The Framingham Heart Study was conducted over sixty years. One of the conclusions was that the state of your lungs will dictate how long you will live. The researchers in this study found that lung capacity can decrease between 9-27% per decade. If you do little or no exercise, and/or you smoke, you could lose 80-90% of your lung capacity by the time you retire. This paints a grim picture for your quality of life. Your lung power is a primary predictor of your health in the future. Even if you have moderate loss, which most people do, your future health is at risk.

The good news is that, regardless of your age, it's not too late to stop the loss, and you can also increase your lung power with the right type of activity.

Your lungs will respond to the right kind of challenge, in the same way your muscles can build strength when they're used. If your exercise routine is based on 'cardio' workouts, you're not challenging your lungs to their full potential. As your body is adaptable it will give up this power, as it's clear you don't need it. Losing your lung power increases your individual ageing process.

Short bursts of high intensity activity challenges your lungs, and over time, your body will adapt to this by increasing your lung capacity and power. It's the same kind of thing that happens to muscles: challenge them and their power grows.

Lung function tests show that people who regularly

exercise in a way that challenges their lungs have 'young lungs', i.e. they have the lung function more typically found in a younger person. They tend to be healthier and slimmer too.

For thousands of years your hunter-gatherer ancestors stayed fit from activities that involved intense exertion, followed by rest. These activities included things like hunting, running and climbing. It kept their bodies lean and muscular. It also kept their lungs in good shape.

Your body is the result of thousands of generations, and as such, you're built for short bursts of intense activity, the same as your ancestors. You build your lungs by challenging them to their maximum capacity. Give it everything you've got for a short period of time then rest, it's that simple.

Looking at the following picture that represents lung function you can see the 'vital capacity'. This represents the total volume of air you can take in, from your lungs feelings empty to them feeling completely full. (Your lungs are never completely empty – you have a 'residual volume' that you can't exhale.) It's your vital capacity that shrinks with age.

It makes sense that if you want to preserve your vital capacity, and hence your lungs, you have to challenge it. How often do you do that? When was the last time you ran as fast as you could? This is the kind of thing your ancestors did most days.

In a typical day, for a typical western person, their breathing stays within the tidal volume. This is how much of your lung capacity you use when relatively inactive. If you go to the gym and do some 'cardio', or go jogging, you will expand your tidal volume, but it's unlikely that you will reach your vital capacity.

Unless you 'work out', your vital capacity will naturally shrink as you get older. Most people do little to change this. A significant number speed it up even more by smoking. But because your body is adaptive, when you 'work out' your vital capacity responds and your lung function improves.

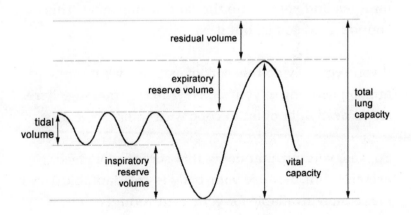

Exercising For Fat Loss

Unless you enjoy all this prolonged cardio workout now is the time to consider ditching it. Let me explain why.

Let's say you're in the gym, jogging on a treadmill or working away on the cross trainer. Your aim is to burn fat. During the first twenty minutes of exercise you will be burning predominantly glucose (not fat), from your glycogen stores. This is just the way your body works. Glycogen is stored in your muscles and liver and is easily broken down into glucose and released into your bloodstream to supply the energy needed for your exercising.

After about twenty minutes of this your body switches from mainly burning glucose to burning predominantly fat instead. Anything over twenty minutes and you're into the fat burning zone. This sounds good so far, but it isn't...

If you regularly do this sort of exercise what message are you sending to your body? The real message here is 'we need a lot of fat to cope with this!'

So, yes, you burn fat doing this sort of prolonged exercise, but because your body is so adaptable it will make more available for your next round.

This is okay if you're happy with your current weight

and you enjoy prolonged exercise on a regular basis
(not many of us do). But if you're not enjoying it,
and it's only holding your weight stable, you may be
scared to stop because you know you'll put weight on.
This is because you've trained your body to make fat
available for the demands you're putting on it.

What Does Your Body Use For Fuel?			
Activity Level	Protein	Carbs	Fat
Resting	1 – 5 %	35%	60%
Low Intensity	5 – 8 %	70 %	15 %
Moderate Intensity	2 – 5 %	40 %	55 %
High Intensity	2 %	95 %	3 %

Adapted from McArdle W, Katch F, Katch V. Sports & Exercise
Nutrition.

New York, NY: Lippincott Williams & Wilkins; 1999

Looking at the chart you can see that low intensity
activity, like walking, derives most of its energy from
glucose. This makes sense because hunter-gatherers
did a lot of this. It's not an activity that encourages fat
storage.

Moderate intensive activity, like jogging, burns fat
more than anything else. This fact inspired people
to exercise at a moderate level and 'cardio' programs
took off. But what really happens here is that you're
training your body to make fat, which is not a good
strategy to lose your body fat! You even burn a greater

percent of fat for your energy needs when you're sat doing nothing compared with jogging. I know which one I prefer.

When it comes to lasting fat loss the most important changes actually happen AFTER exercise, NOT during exercise. Short bursts of high intensity exercise use nearly all glucose. This tells your body that storing a load of energy as fat isn't the thing it needs. It needs loads of energy stored in your muscles because that's where most of your energy is coming from. Because your body is adaptable it will learn to store more energy as glucose, and less as fat.

I Haven't Got Time To Exercise!

If you're not doing any exercise because you think you haven't got time, based on what you know about cardio, then it's good news - that reason will no longer be relevant to you any longer.

Considering our genes haven't changed in tens of thousands of years, good information about great ways to exercise can be gleaned for our ancestors, and those that still live like them today.

Hunter-gatherers tend to do quite a lot of walking, and they also do regular brief bouts of explosive activity, e.g. running to catch things or running away from things.

These brief bouts of maximal exertion use a lot of glucose from your glycogen stores. But you're interested in fat burning, right? Your body is very adaptable, which means whatever you regularly do, your body will change to serve that requirement better. If you regularly run long distances your body will store fat to cope with this. This fat will start making an appearance if you have a week or two off.

Taking a leaf out of the hunter-gatherer book, they don't do 'cardio' exercise. Why would they? That would be a waste of energy, and time. They don't go into the 'fat burning zone' with their 'exercise' - they remain in the glucose burning zone.

So what happens if you limit your exercise to short bouts squeezed into just twenty minutes or less? Because your body is adaptable it's going to learn to store more energy, as glycogen, in your liver and muscles. Glycogen is easily accessible and breaks down into glucose quickly when you exercise. This means less fat storage. Fat takes longer to get back out into your circulation, and your body now requires lots of energy fast, but only for 20 minutes at a time – not long enough to get your fat reserves out into your bloodstream, therefore, you don't need to store so much.

When you do 'fat burning cardio' exercise you burn fat while you're doing it, but once you finish, this fat burning quickly tails off.

When you exercise at a high rate for a short period of time and push yourself towards your maximum, your body has to work hard to repair and restore itself afterwards. It takes a LOT of calories to do this. Depending on how much you've exerted yourself, it can take up to a full day for your body to complete this work. The energy to do this mostly comes mainly from fat, and is known as the 'after burn'.

With extended workouts, e.g. jogging, your fat burning tails off quickly once you stop. You are, in effect, training your body to store fat for the next bout. It's an inefficient way to try and lose your body fat, to say the very least.

With short, high intensity workouts you don't burn much fat while you're doing it, but you do afterwards. Fat burning can go on for up to a day after you've had a maximal workout. You'll have spent twenty minutes, or less, and still be burning fat hours after. I'd call that a pretty efficient way to lose your body fat. It also blows the most common reason or excuse for not exercising - 'I haven't got time' - completely out of the water.

24. Your 20-minute Exercise Plan

If your sole purpose of exercise is to lose fat, or you

feel like you haven't got time to exercise, this is the way forward for you. If you love endurance exercise, like jogging, there's no need to stop that. However, you will benefit hugely by incorporating short, high intensity exercise into your routine. This will benefit your heart and lung health as well as speed up your fat loss.

It doesn't matter what your starting point of fitness is, because you start at your own individual level. However, you've got to be sensible and check with your doctor before starting this if any of the following apply to you:

- **Over 50 years old and no exercise for years**
- **No kind of medical check for two years or more**
- **High blood pressure that isn't under control**
- **Any heart problem**
- **Family history of heart attacks before 60 years old**
- **Any lung problem**
- **More than 2 stone (28lb) overweight**

If you haven't exercised for years it's important to start slow and gradually increase over time. This isn't a race - there's no rush, just steady progress.

Here's a blog entry I wrote about exercise:

If you're exercising and not losing weight, chances are you're doing the wrong sort of exercise for effective weight loss.

Some years ago, researchers in Canada took two groups of people and gave them two different exercise programmes to follow.

The first group had the conventional 'fat burning' type of exercise and they had to cycle for 45 minutes, uninterrupted. The second group had to do short bursts of cycling for 15-90 seconds, with rests in-between.

The group that did the continuous 45 minute cycle burned more calories than the group doing the interval-style exercise. In fact, they burned twice as many calories. No surprise there.

You would think, therefore, that the first group would have burned more fat – not so! In fact, the group doing the short bursts of exercise burned nine times more fat for each calorie burned, compared to the long cycle group.

How can this be right?

*People tend to focus on what is happening **during** exercise and ignore what happens **after** the exercise has finished. In a nutshell, interval-like exercise causes more fat burning after the exercise has taken place.*

In direct contrast, the 45 minute cycling moved

participants' bodies into the 'fat burning zone' while they were doing it, but when this is done repeatedly it teaches your body it needs fat available for the next round of prolonged exercise. You end up just replacing what you've used.

If you're not keen on exercise, and are only doing it to be healthier and to lose weight, do yourself a favour and learn how to do it so it works for you, rather than against you.

I like things to be as quick and as easy as possible but still get great results. Unless you like it, life is too short to spend loads of time exercising!

So how do you put this into practice to build your health AND lose fat? You're going to exercise intensely and get your heart rate right up, but you're going to limit your workouts to twenty minutes, or less. You're going to focus on brief bouts of significant exertion broken up with slower paced activity. The slower pace is to give your heart rate recovery time.

If you don't currently do any exercise at all, and are a self-confessed couch potato, this may be your starting point. If you're really out of shape, or haven't done anything to get your heart rate up for years, start off walking at a reasonable pace, but not enough to be properly out of breath. Once you've warmed up, after about five minutes, pick up the pace to a fast walk.

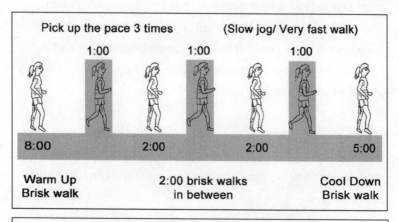

Pick up the pace 3 times   (Slow jog/ Very fast walk)

1:00   1:00   1:00

8:00   2:00   2:00   5:00

Warm Up   2:00 brisk walks   Cool Down
Brisk walk   in between   Brisk walk

LIGHT INTERVAL TRAINING:
A 20 minute Walk- Jog Workout

This should be fast enough to make you out of breath after a minute. Now slow down to catch your breath for two minutes. Repeat this two more times and then finish with a five-minute cool down walk.

When you've done this a few times, and are getting comfortable with it, it's time to pick things up a bit. What you're really aiming for is to be properly out of breath after you've finished your minute of exertion. At the end you should be panting and having to take in big lungfuls of air to get your breath back. When you reach this state you're challenging your lungs and really working your muscles. You're doing your general health a great service, and you'll have put in a great effort towards your fat loss aim.

When this stops being a challenge, or if it isn't in the

first place, do a slow jog instead of fast walking. Or you could power-walk up an incline. As you progress, this will get easier, so take a step up again. Some more examples are coming up. Taking a step up demonstrates increased lung power which is amazing for your overall health.

You can walk straight out of your front door and be back in twenty minutes. You can do this with a pushchair, or a little kiddie on a bike next to you, if you've got little children with you all day. You could incorporate this during a walk to work or just to the shops. If you've got a dog, do it while walking him/her. Or this could just be your time out for twenty minutes.

If walking and/or jogging is not your thing there are plenty of other ways to do this:
- Running – either outside or on a treadmill
- Swimming
- Cycling – either outside or on an exercise bike
- Running on the spot on a rebounder (mini trampoline)
- Any exercise machine at the gym

With different sorts of exercise just slow your pace right down in-between bouts of really pushing yourself. You definitely don't need to go to a gym to do this, but if you enjoy going to the gym, continue to do so.

This type of exercise increases the fitness and health of your heart and lungs, which is a brilliant thing to do. It also increases your muscle mass, which is going to help with your fat loss efforts too.

When the first plan is too easy, or you are fitter than that, it's time to up your game. Here's an example of a step up:

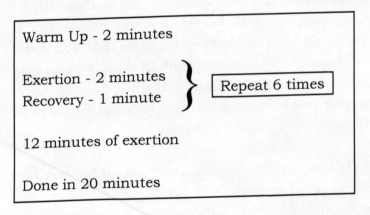

If six repetitions is too much for you, start at four; as you get fitter, increase it. The idea is to pack as much as you can into the time you're exercising. There's no need to go over twenty minutes, because if you do, you're into the fat burning zone (and you definitely don't need to be here to lose fat). You don't even have to do twenty minutes. Here's another example:

```
Warm Up - 5 minutes

Exertion - 20 seconds  }
                        }  [ Repeat 6 times ]
Recovery - 60 seconds  }

2 minutes of exertion

Done in 13 minutes
```

On the face of it, the one you can do in thirteen minutes might look easier. That's not the case. The idea is, when doing your bout of exercise, you should do as much as you can in that time - so if you're doing a twenty-second bout of exercise you'll be going a lot faster than if you were doing a two-minute bout. Just think of the exertion a two hundred metre sprinter puts into a race – that's about twenty seconds. So don't choose this one for the easy option! It's great, however, if you don't have a lot of time to spare.

It's best not to stick to one exercise plan because your body just gets used to it, and it consequently becomes less challenging. Without any challenge you won't be pushing your lungs and muscles to their maximum. This means you won't be making any progress and you risk slipping backwards. Mixing it up also prevents you from getting bored.

One day, concentrate on bouts of exercise that take a

couple of minutes; another day, do something quicker and shorter. Here are some more examples, but you can create your own too, to suit you. All you need to incorporate are a few essential things:

- Keep your workout to twenty minutes or less
- Start off with a small warm up
- Have repeated bouts of maximal exertion, followed by recovery time
- If you don't feel really out of breath at the end, you haven't achieved very much, because this means you haven't challenged your lungs or muscles enough for what you're aiming to do, i.e. lose fat and increase your health

Warm Up - 5 minutes

Exertion - 4 minutes
Rest - 1 minute
Exertion - 3 minutes
Rest - 1 minute
Exertion - 2 minutes
Rest - 1 minute
Exertion - 1 minute
Recovery - 2 minute

Done in 20 minutes

Warm Up - 5 minutes

Exertion - 1 minute - Recovery 30 seconds
Exertion - 1 minute - Recovery 30 seconds
Exertion - 30 seconds - Recovery 30 seconds
Exertion - 20 seconds - Recovery 30 seconds
Exertion - 20 seconds - Recovery 30 seconds

Done!

This is all about working harder and smarter for less time. This is a great investment towards your health and fat loss, for minimal time input. You only need to do this about three times a week to turbo charge your health and fat loss. That's a maximum of an hour a week. To get even more benefit you can combine this with a bit or strength work too (coming next). You don't need to start all of this at the same time. Perhaps start with the twenty-minute workouts and when they become part of your routine look at adding in some strength work too.

25. Building A Bit Of Muscle

Hunter-gatherers do short bouts of strenuous activity, and you've got that bit covered now. They also do activity that builds and maintains muscle strength. You burn most of your calories in your muscles, so the more muscle you've got, the more calories you burn. Remember: you lose muscle by going on a restrictive diet, so avoid these from now on at all costs.

It's best to start with building your heart and lung strength, from high exertion exercise. You will build some muscle strength by doing this, but ideally, you need to do a bit more for the most benefit.

The typical western environment causes the same problem for your muscles as it does for your lungs. It doesn't provide the strength challenges your body is designed for. Mother Nature has designed your body to build and maintain muscle in response to the demands associated with your own body weight. Think about a hunter-gatherer climbing or jumping. They didn't use machines or weights to develop their bodies.

Moving your own body weight is the most effective way to build your strength. You don't need any specialised equipment or a gym to do it.

You will not become all muscle-bound by doing these activities. A bit of muscle makes your body look nicer – it pulls your belly and your bum in, adds shape, and brings definition to your arms and legs.

Yoga

My main choice of strength exercise is yoga. If you've
not done yoga before you really have to do it to
appreciate how much strength it takes. I started it
because I was getting stiff and had a few persistent
aches and pains, like back pain, tight Achilles
tendons and shoulder stiffness. My posture wasn't
great and was probably causing my back pain. I
thought yoga would help with all of this but it still
took me months and months to take the first step and
start going. If I had known how much I would come to
love it and the great effect it had on my body I would
have gone years ago.

Within just ten weeks of starting most of my aches
and pains had gone, and I had flexibility I didn't even
have as a teenager. But the thing that really delighted
me was how it pulled my waist and rear end in. I
didn't lose any weight (I didn't need to at this time),
but my clothes looked better. My body felt generally
firmer.

The other huge benefit of yoga is that it teaches you
to switch off your thoughts and tune into your body.
This is not only hugely relaxing for your mind at the
time, but it also helps you become more aware of the
sensations in your body and mind generally. This
helps you tune into your hunger and any emotions
that may be driving you to eat, and is particularly

helpful if you're a comfort eater.

In a nutshell I can't recommend yoga highly enough. Consider giving it a go, but give it a chance, because when you first start it can feel quite hard. The thing to do with yoga, like all things worth doing, is to take it at your own pace. Don't look at your teacher, or people who have been going for years, and feel disheartened, because you can't do what they do. They were rubbish at it when they started too. I'd recommend going at least twice a week.

Other Strength Exercises

If yoga isn't for you, or if it's not going to fit in with your schedule, there are other things you can do at home that don't take long.

I appreciate time is a real issue for a lot of people. Here's a blog I wrote in January 2014.

How to Start Exercising

'I have no time to exercise!'; 'I hate exercise!'; 'Even the thought of exercise feels like hard work, let alone doing it!'

These are just a few of the more polite things one of my clients had to say to me about exercise. However, she also recognised that it was only by doing some that she would achieve her aim of being fit and healthy.

Jane is a busy lady in her late forties who works full time in an office-based job. When we first spoke she was too tired to do any exercise after work and had no intention of getting up early to do any. Fair enough.

So, where do you start?

Your muscles are a key player in keeping you slim and keeping you healthy so they're a good place to start. This is what Jane started with.

- **5 'girly' push ups before going to work**
- **10 squats when she visited the ladies' room mid-morning, while at work**
- **20 seconds of a modified plank when she got home from work**

Quite easily Jane solved her problem of how to start exercising. What she'd done was make a start! The push ups built upper body muscle, the plank built core strength and muscle, and the squats built lower body muscle.

This very basic, simple, and quick work out is a great start for people who think they haven't got time to exercise. It also gets over the problem of it being too hard.

I know Jane has gradually increased where she

started from. Each week she increased how many squats and press ups she did. She became strong enough to do 'proper press ups'. She gradually increased how long she held her modified plank and built up to doing a full one. Later, she added some different exercises.

You can see just how easy it is to solve the problem of 'how to start exercising'. This takes hardly any time or effort, so get started!

Before I started yoga my strength exercises included the ones below. I would do these three times a week and it would take me about ten minutes.

1. For your core – the plank

Lie on the floor, face-down, and then lift yourself onto your elbows and forearms and your toes. When you're in the correct position your body is completely straight (like a plank of wood). Make sure your bum isn't poking up in the air or dropping down. Hold this position for as long as you can. If you've never done this before you might not even manage 30 seconds; that's okay.

You could aim to add an extra five seconds every week or two to make sure you're getting better and you're continuing to develop muscle strength.

This exercise is great for pulling your stomach in. Because it strengthens your core it also helps any back pain you may have.

If this is too difficult to do, start it on your knees until you are strong enough to do the full version. Make sure you keep your body in a straight line from your knees.

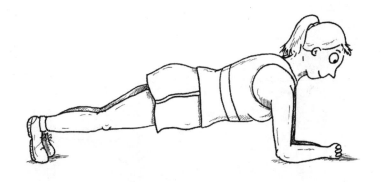

2. For your legs – squats

Having good strength to do this one as you get older is really important. It exercises the biggest muscle groups in your body: your thighs, hamstrings and glutes (the muscles in your bum). It's keeping strength here that allows you to get up out of a chair. One of the things that can rob people of their independence is not being able to do this.

Stand with your feet shoulder width apart. Keeping the weight mainly going through your heels, bend your knees and your hips to right angles. Keep your back straight. This movement is like sitting down in a chair. Stand back up again.

Just do ten the first time you do it. As the weeks go on, gradually increase it. One of my clients gradually built up to a hundred over quite a few months, so this gives her heart and lungs a good work out too at the same time.

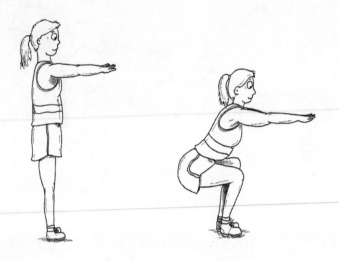

3. For your upper body, core and arms - press ups

Lie down with your palms on the floor next to your shoulders. Have the balls of your feet on the ground. Keep your body straight and lift your body up until your arms are straight.

Lower yourself down until your elbows reach a

90-degree angle and then push yourself up again.

If this is too hard, start on your knees. It's important
to keep your body straight. See how many you can do,
it might not be many at all when you first start; this is
fine. Gradually build up as the weeks go on.
When I first did these I could just squeeze out one
before collapsing! I just stuck with doing one of each
of the workouts until I could do it without bursting
a blood vessel. I then increased up to two, and as I
gradually got stronger, built up from there.

The important thing is not to think you're achieving
very little if you can only do one girly push up on your
knees before you're done in. This is just your starting
point. It's only your patience that will get you beyond
this.

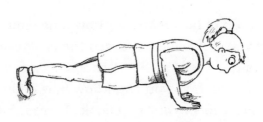

4. For your upper body and arms – dips

Get a chair, bend your knees and put your hands on
the seat of the chair. Bend your elbows to 90 degrees
so your body lowers down. Push yourself back up
using your arms (not your legs).

Again, see how many you can do on your first time.
Stick with this number for a week or two and then
gradually start adding more.

I deliberately kept this short and sweet because I
think this is a good start, and you can make a lot
of progress with just these four exercises. Aim to do
them about three times a week.

This type of exercise challenges your muscles close
to their peak, so you build strength and muscle.
You only need to do a few so you can get this done
really fast. Because you're working muscles in groups
(rather than isolated muscles on a machine in the
gym) this increases your efficiency; you get results in
a short amount of time. Exercising this way is also
more natural for your body.

Keep a record of how many, or how long, you can do.
This way you can see for yourself the progress you're
making as the weeks go by. Perhaps keep a record
of when you do it, so you can know how often you're
doing it. Put this in your notebook. Things that get

measured tend to get done.

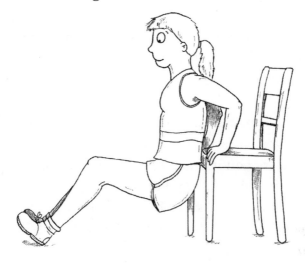

26. Putting It All Together

You have hunter-gatherer genes, so how can you tie all of this together to have the same fitness (and slimness) in today's 21st century western world?

Ideally, your foundation is plenty of light activity. An average of 10,000 steps is a really good level to aim for. This would be taken from the moment you got up to when you go back to bed. It includes all of your steps, even if it's just to the loo.

You could consider getting a pedometer (a little gadget that measures how many steps you take) to see where you're at now and see how far off the mark you are. If you are way under look at ways you can gradually increase it. This can be so easy: taking the stairs; walking short distances instead of taking the car; not parking the car as close to the front door as possible; taking a short walk in your breaks at work instead of sitting, drinking coffee.

Note I said *gradually*. Don't rush to make any big changes with regards to activity and exercise. Chances are you will get fed up quickly and stop. Start slow and build up. Perhaps aim to increase your baseline number of steps by 2,000 for a while. Once this new level feels normal increase it a bit more.

Getting your daily average steps up is a brilliant place to start. You could perhaps write something in your notebook about your intentions regarding this.

If you already do quite a lot of walking, or you're looking to be a bit more active, start experimenting with some interval training. Again, start slowly and build up. Your aim with this is to get yourself panting and really out of breath. If you can only manage to do two repetitions on your first attempt, that's okay. You'll get better, don't be disheartened.

The first time I tried this I chose sprinting. At the time I thought I was pretty fit and I wasn't carrying excess weight to slow me down. I managed three and a half reps of about 30 seconds each. I had planned on doing six, but that didn't happen – I was completely done in. My starting point with this particular routine, therefore, was one minute and 45 seconds of exercise! However, my heart and lungs had a great workout, and my leg muscles obviously had too, because they barely got me home. This soon got better.

Start incorporating some strength exercises. You could even just start with one of these. For example, you might choose squats. You could do this two or three times a week for a while and then add in another exercise. Make this easy on yourself, there's never any need to make life difficult by rushing.

Don't go mad with exercise. If you've done an interval-style training session, and you've really tired yourself out, it's a good idea to have the next day off from anything heavy.

In summary, the ideal exercise plan would look something like this:
- Plenty of low intensity activity, like walking (build up to an average of 10,000 steps/day – perhaps get a pedometer to keep track of how well you're doing)
- Regular short bursts of high intensity activity
  - to challenge your heart and lungs, e.g. fast walking, or running when you're fitter – 3 times per week is more than enough
  - to challenge your muscles to close to their maximum, i.e. a bit of strength work – 2- 3

times per week
- 1 or 2 rest days

If you haven't done any exercise for ages begin by increasing your daily steps – this is a good place to start in your position. Remember, this is about you, nobody else. You're not in competition with anyone, only yourself. The competition with yourself involves gradually improving on your previous performance.

Then gradually build in the other kinds of exercise as you get a bit fitter. Your aim is to make steady progress. Record what you're doing in your notebook so you can check up on yourself – the aim is progress, not repeating the same thing week in, week out.

Part 5 – Metabolism
27. Introduction

This part really starts pulling the strands together, regarding what you eat and what you do. It reinforces the message that you have to become healthy to get the body you're after. It can't be done with fad diets.

Research shows that the major factor in people's longevity, and perhaps more importantly, the quality of their life, is down to their muscle mass. Your muscle mass has everything to do with your metabolism. Other things related to your metabolism include:

- The amount of body fat you have
- The strength of your immune system
- Skin wrinkles
- Joint pain
- Memory loss

Studies of identical twins have shown that around 35% of the ageing process is down to genetics (which is out of your control). But that means the other 65% is in your hands. Metabolism, not genetics, is the primary factor that influences how fast (or slow) your body ages, and most of it you have control over.

There's constant dialogue between your brain and your body and this is a big determining factor regarding how you age and when you will die.

When the brain receives 'longevity signals' from a healthy body it sends messages back that make sure the body is well maintained and kept in good shape. This body still has a lot to give.

When things start to slide in the body, the brain receives 'over-the-hill' signals instead. As a result the brain sends back very different signals, and these start the slow breakdown of your body. It assumes this body hasn't much left to give.

To appreciate why this happens you only need to look at Mother Nature. Humans are far too wrapped up in themselves and often forget they are just a small part of Mother Nature.

Mother Nature is concerned with the survival of the species. Individuals don't matter to her as she is only interested in the bigger picture. As an individual you're insignificant and on your own.

The genes you have today are the same as your ancestors had 30,000 years ago. The program in your genes causes your brain to shift into a slow breakdown if the body isn't sending regular signals to the brain that it's in good shape. This is why most common illnesses strike people as they get older; it's all part of the breakdown process.

When your muscle activity is low, this is a very bad

sign to your brain. Instructions are hardwired into your genes to initiate the slow shutdown process. You have a body that's designed to be used, it is carved indelibly into your genes. If your body isn't used sufficiently then your brain assumes something is very wrong. To Mother Nature you aren't really useful to the survival of the species anymore; it's nothing personal, it was fun while it lasted, but you're not useful now and she needs to make way for someone new.

Think about that the next time you're sat on the sofa munching on some processed rubbish in front of the TV. You think you're having fun and being entertained, but if this is your routine the biochemical readout from your body back to your brain paints a grim picture. Your brain hears:

- Poor muscle mass
- Muscles not being used
- Inactive
- Excess body fat
- Unproductive body

Breakdown signals go back to your body, which results in you getting sick and dying earlier than you should. And many of the years before your early death will not be much fun for you.

Today's technology is making people arrogant towards Mother Nature, to their peril. The average life expectancy in the UK is 81 years. But most people end up suffering all sorts of illness, which are preventable.

I find it interesting that, on average, nearly every mammal lives at least ten times longer than their age at puberty. Humans manage six to seven times their age at puberty. And we are the only ones who mess with their food and often shun what Mother Nature provides.

This indifference to Mother Nature has people reaching for caffeine when they feel fatigued, going on diets to lose weight (or worse, taking pills). This works against your genetic makeup and sends more damaging signals back to your brain.

In a nutshell, your chances of getting slim, and keeping it that way, are few, if you don't restore your healthy metabolism.

What you consistently do in terms of your eating, drinking and exercise shapes your metabolism. Are you beginning to see just how important all of this stuff is?

As well as heavily influencing your weight you also know that your metabolism determines how healthy you are and how long you will live. This is really serious stuff.

Quality of life (in terms of health) tends to rise through childhood, and you enjoy a peak of good health between the ages of 15-35 years old. These are usually the prime years of your life when it comes to your health.

But then the downward slope begins as people start to experience degeneration of their body. This may show up as high blood pressure, diabetes, arthritis, heart disease, cancer, and many other health problems. When you don't look after your metabolism this is what your life is likely to be like. Maybe you feel 'over the hill' already.

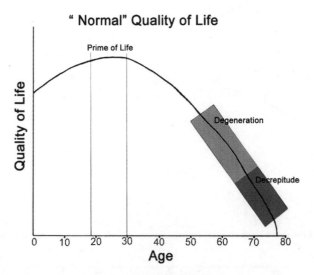

It doesn't have to be like this, though, even if you feel that you're already on the downward slope. By restoring your healthy metabolism you can either stay on a high with your health (and ideal weight) for many more years or you can restore yourself to good health and your ideal weight. Going back to the rat experiment, it's possible to do something about this, even if you feel well over the hill.

There is a population of people, known as the Hunzas, who live in the foothills of the Himalayas. They continue to live a primitive life. There's a lot of interest in these people because they tend to live so long. It's not unusual for them to live well beyond 100, and in good health too. Much of this is thought to be due to good nutrition and an active lifestyle (nothing to do with western living and modern medicine). This really makes you think.

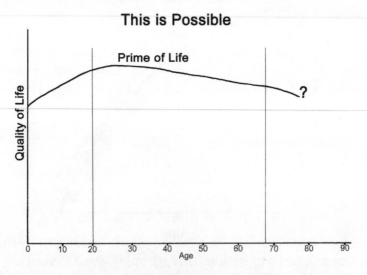

Many people think their metabolism is all about how fast they burn up calories. Whilst it is to do with this, it is also about so much more.

There are two sides to the metabolic coin, and they work in opposite directions.

You have your anabolic metabolism. This is all to do with:
• Repairing, rebuilding and restoring your body
• Fat burning

You also have your catabolic metabolism. This is the opposite, and it's involved in:
• Breakdown and degeneration of your body
• Fat storage

Your health and weight are determined by the ratio of these two.

If you're thinking you want to increase you anabolic metabolism and decrease your catabolic metabolism you're on the right lines, and that's essentially what this part is all about.

28. How Is Your Metabolism Determined?

There is constant communication happening within your body from one part to another via hormones. One small circuit of this communication involves your brain being in contact with your digestive track and your muscles.

Your muscles play a key role when it comes to this

three-way communication. If your routine is pretty inactive and your muscle mass is fairly low, your brain gets the message that very little energy is required, simply because you aren't burning up very much.

So, your brain gets the message that little energy is required. When you eat, the hormonal message from your brain to your stomach will be something like this: 'convert these calories to fat because this body doesn't currently need them for energy'. You put weight on.

If, conversely, you are *regularly* active and have a higher muscle mass, the message is going to be very different. This time, the message from your brain to your digestive track is 'convert these calories to energy because this body is active and needs them'. You won't put weight on, or you start to lose it.

This continuous hormonal dialogue between your muscles, brain and digestive track also contributes to your overall health. An active and vibrant body sends healthy longevity signals to your brain. Your brain sends healthy maintenance signals back. If you want to enjoy good health for a long time you need to look after your metabolism by eating right and moving your body.

Hormonal signals between your brain and your body

are, in effect, your 'longevity signals':

- Your brain receives healthy longevity signals from your body (largely from your muscles) → your brain sends anabolic (repair and rebuild) instructions back to your body, *including burning fat.*

- Your brain receives 'over the hill' signals from your body (because you don't have a lot of muscle mass and are doing other things to damage your metabolism) → your brain sends catabolic (breakdown) instructions back, which encourages the *laying down of fat.*

There's far more to your metabolism than simply how fast or slow you burn calories.

Let's learn how to put the brakes on your catabolic activity and reduce the amount of fat you store. Then you'll find out how to restore your anabolic metabolism that will see you burning fat and increasing your energy levels.

Little of this will be brand new; you've covered a lot of this already. But you will see how your food and exercise choices influence your metabolism, and hence, the amount of fat you store.

29. Putting The Brakes On Catabolic Metabolism

A lot of the information you've learned so far will be

starting to fit together. To slow down the catabolic signals travelling around your body there are three things to consider:

- Reducing the damaging effect of free radicals on your body
- Reducing the amount of glucose damage (glycation) within your body
- Reducing the damage inflicted on your liver

If some of these terms have gone straight over your head all will become clear as you read on.

Free Radicals

When you drive your car you burn petrol. There are good and bad consequences from burning petrol. The good is that the energy created enables you to drive your car and travel to places. The bad is the exhaust fumes released into the atmosphere, which damages the environment.

When you burn things within your body, like glucose and fatty acids for energy, oxygen is used in the process and energy is produced. This is very similar to the petrol in your car. The energy produced is the good effect. Unfortunately, there's a bad effect too: free radical formation. And just as exhaust fumes from your car are an unwanted but necessary consequence, so too are free radicals within your body.

Free radicals are one of the major reasons your body ages; they cause wrinkles on your skin and cause your body to deteriorate and get older. They do this by latching onto healthy tissues and damaging them. Within the skin they attach to the proteins elastin and collagen. Over time these proteins change from being quite elastic and stretchy to being stiff and inflexible.

The downside of energy production within your body is the creation of free radicals. Although this is normal, your body needs to be properly equipped to deal with these. Otherwise, the free radicals will harm you by causing damage to healthy cells and tissues.

What's the result of free radical damage?

If free radicals go unchecked and are allowed to run rampage through your body, you will succumb to at least one of the degenerative diseases that are common in affluent western countries. These include:

- heart disease
- stroke
- dementia
- cancer
- arthritis
- skin wrinkles (not a disease, but certainly not desirable)

You need a lot of antioxidants to combat all of these free radicals, and you get a lot of them from what you eat - or at least you should.

What are antioxidants?

Antioxidants act like scavengers. They seek out free radicals and neutralise them before they're able to do their damage. There are thousands of different antioxidants, some of which are produced in your body. However, you need to eat a good amount of food containing antioxidants to have enough to neutralise the free radicals you produce constantly. Examples of antioxidants are the vitamins C, E, and folic acid.

Fresh fruit and vegetables (more so, organic) are great sources of antioxidants, and this is one reason why they're ESSENTIAL to your daily diet. They provide the building blocks to your body to defend itself against free radical attack.

As pointed out before, it's also important how you prepare them. You will get the full benefit from eating them raw, where appropriate. If you want to cook, the best way to preserve as many of the goodies as possible is by steaming. Using a microwave will destroy just about all of the goodness in any fresh food.

Ongoing free radical damage taking place throughout your body is not good at all, and results in catabolic messages being sent to your brain. This adds to the downward health spiral you might be on. Catabolic signals go hand in hand with fat storage too.

To put the brakes on this sort of catabolic activity, eat plenty of antioxidant rich food:

- Fresh fruit and vegetables, every day
- Fruit – berries are particularly good
- Fresh vegetables – dark green are best, like kale, spinach, broccoli
- Eat as much of these as possible, either raw or steamed
- Consider juicing fruit and vegetables
- Raw nuts and seeds
- Beans
- Oily fish – sardine, mackerel, salmon

This is all about increasing antioxidants. When it comes to fruit and vegetables you'll get more benefit from organically grown. This is because lower levels of antioxidants are found in 'normal' produce due to modern methods of farming. Unfortunately, due to intensive farming methods, much of the soil has been stripped of nutrients, therefore the produce is deficient too.

It's better to have organic because you get more nutrients and fewer chemicals, by way of pesticides.

Going back to the rat experiment you can begin to see why the ones fed a healthy and antioxidant rich diet did so well. Remember, those who were fed the rubbish diet reversed health and weight problems by having a healthy one.

Glucose Damage

You need glucose in your bloodstream, but only relatively low levels. Because of the diet our ancestors ate their levels were likely to be lower than what's considered normal today. There are good reasons to keep your blood glucose levels relatively low. A certain amount of glucose in your bloodstream is necessary, but unfortunately, it does your body harm too.

You need glucose circulating in your bloodstream, but it naturally combines with proteins in your body and damages them. This process is known as glycation. This is a slow process and eventually shows up as things like wrinkles on your face and by the hardening of your arteries, which can end up in heart attacks and strokes. The more glucose you allow into your system, the faster this will happen, i.e. the faster you'll age. This ends up sending a load of catabolic signals around your body.

Remember, lots of catabolic activity is really bad for you and *makes you more likely to store fat.*

So, how do you slow glycation damage down?

Every time you eat things that are absorbed as glucose by your body, you cause glycation. To a certain extent, this is inevitable. But the quicker food releases its glucose, the higher your blood glucose rises. The more glucose that's around the more opportunity it has to combine with proteins and damage them. Another example of this damage is cataracts. Glucose has combined with the proteins in the lens of the eye, changing it from clear to opaque.

It's a good idea to keep your portion sizes down when it comes to carbs, filling up with vegetables instead. You particularly want to keep to a minimum these kinds of things:
- Sugar
- Refined carbs
- Most conventional wheat products (pasta is okay)

Going back to the unlucky rats that were fed a lifetime of processed refined rubbish, they suffered a huge amount of this type of damage, in addition to the free radical damage. These two things go pretty much hand in hand, and over many years, have catastrophic effect on health.

Looking After Your Liver

Your liver is your main detoxifier. It keeps your internal system running smoothly by sorting out and making safe just about everything that comes into your body. It keeps your body clean and healthy.

A healthy liver is essential to a good anabolic metabolism, a metabolism that has you feeling full of energy and burning fat, rather than storing it. A weakened liver sends catabolic signals to your brain, which speeds up catabolic metabolism. This means you age faster and lay down fat.

This is one of the reasons why heavy drinkers age quickly. They put a lot of strain on their liver and, as a result, shift their balance heavily towards catabolic metabolism and away from anabolic.

These days, a common form of injury to the liver is fatty infiltration. This is when fat is stored within internal organs as well as under the skin. Many people think their fat is just under the surface, looking unsightly. I'm afraid it's more sinister than that. The more excess pounds you carry, the more likely you are to have a fatty liver. But as you lose your excess fat this will correct itself.

When it comes to liver health, it's really important to get enough good sleep. When you get good quality sleep, which includes the deep restorative kind, your body does a lot of repair work. This is the time your liver does much of its own maintenance and, depending on how you've treated it, it might really need it.

Sometimes, people are their own worst enemies when it comes to getting enough sleep. But other times you could be inadvertently wrecking the quality of your sleep.

You already know it's quite hard to get your full complement of deep sleep when you drink caffeine regularly. In addition to wrecking your sleep caffeine has to be broken down, otherwise it would just build up in your body and you would be permanently wired. Your liver has the job of breaking caffeine down to make it harmless and to rid it from your body. Your liver is good at doing this, but it could probably get on with better work, like restoring your anabolic metabolism.

Caffeine also pushes you towards catabolic metabolism by dehydrating you and causing your adrenal glands to release stress hormones into your system.

You don't necessarily have to stop caffeine altogether, but think about what you're doing to yourself when you choose to drink it. Perhaps just have it when you're really going to enjoy it and appreciate it, rather than just out of habit, because you're not thinking.

Another thing that can interfere with your sleep is a diet high in refined carbs and sugar. You already know that this 'food' is no good for your waistline, but besides disrupting your sleep, it has the knock-on effect of pushing you towards catabolic metabolism too. Refined food plays havoc with your hormones, particularly your stress hormones from your adrenal glands.

Alcohol is the obvious liver toxin. Everyone knows that too much alcohol is bad for your liver. But not everyone knows that too much will push your metabolism towards the catabolic side of the equation.

It takes an enormous amount of work and effort for your liver to break alcohol down. It has to do this because alcohol is seen by your body as a toxin that has to be made safe as soon as possible. Other work will be put on the back burner until the alcohol problem is dealt with. And while your liver is dealing with alcohol, it's being taken away from its other work - restoring your anabolic metabolism.

Don't worry, I'm not suggesting you join the temperance society and become teetotal!

The recommendations we have in the UK regarding safe alcohol consumption are fairly sensible I think:
- 14 units per week for women, and no more than 2-3 units in a day
- 21 units per week for men and no more than 3-4 units in a day
- Have two or three alcohol-free days

The difference between men and women is largely down to the fact that men have bigger livers, because they're generally bigger than women. This means men generally have a bigger liver capacity so they can deal with higher levels of alcohol before it causes them damage. A woman trying to keep up with a man while drinking is not doing herself any favours at all, and will lose the health game in the long run.

Even these recommendations might be too much for you, so it's important to listen to your body.

Another way to reduce the strain on your liver is to eat organic food when possible. Non-organic foods will have pesticides on and/or within them. Pesticides are designed to kill things so there is no way they can be beneficial to a human body. In my opinion having 'safe levels' of these chemicals in our food is nonsense. How can things made to kill be safe for us to eat?

Your liver has to break these chemicals down to make them non-harmful to your body. They also need breaking down so they can be eliminated from your body. This is yet another strain on your liver, distracting it from pushing towards an anabolic, fat burning metabolism.

If you're not eating organic fruit and vegetables, give them a really good scrub to get as many chemicals off as possible.

Over the counter medications, prescription drugs and recreational drugs all add to your liver's work. These are all detoxified and broken down by your liver. Check with your doctor if you're not convinced you need all the tablets you may be on. This is a really good reason to only take the medication that's essential.

To recap, the things to do to look after your liver involve:

- Getting enough good quality sleep
- Losing excess body fat
- Reducing, or even eliminating, caffeine
- Reducing to a minimum sugar and refined carbs
- Being sensible with alcohol
- Eating more organic food
- Keeping medication use to a minimum

Generally, this supports your liver and helps push the scales towards a healthy, fat burning, anabolic metabolism. Your liver will love you when you reduce the assaults you inflict on it. It can concentrate instead on restoring your metabolism.

30. How To Improve Your Anabolic Metabolism

A lot of this won't be new, you've been learning about this right from the start.

Gain Muscle

Sometimes women worry when I advise they increase their muscle mass that they're going to look unfeminine. Women can have more than enough muscle mass without looking muscle-bound. In fact, if you're a woman, you'll have to work very hard to look muscly! Men put on muscle mass more easily.

In short, more muscle mass means:
- more fat burning capability
- more energy for you
- better shape to your body
- lots of lovely anabolic signals to your brain, which, in turn, give anabolic (including fat burning) signals back to your body

It's so important that you never do a restrictive diet again. Restrictive diets lead to muscle loss before you lose any fat. This just encourages catabolic metabolism and reduces your fat burning capacity. Once you're eating better you will have more energy to make a start on your exercise routine. But there's no rush, start slow and gradually improve as it gets easier.

Nutrition

A healthy metabolism can only exist if you give your body the raw materials it needs to build one. These obviously come from the food you choose to eat.

A correctly functioning metabolism burns fat to create energy rather than storing it and making you feel sluggish.

Most of this was covered in part 3, but in a nutshell, it involves:

- Eating whole, unrefined foods – real food that hasn't been mucked about with
- Eating a wide variety of foods – this gives a good range of the smaller nutrients
- Eating plenty of fruit and vegetables every day, some of them raw
- Eating good quality meat and fish (if this is part of your diet)
- Hydrating yourself well with eight glasses of water per day

Some people are concerned about the cost of eating healthy food. I do understand this concern; however, when you gradually change your diet to healthy, nutritious food you'll notice you don't eat quite so much. This is because your appetite is no longer being driven by unnatural foods. This balances the cost to a large extent.

Remember, there's no rush with this.

Good Digestion

In addition to *what* you eat, *how* you eat is really

important too.

Some of this will probably sound like complete common sense, and you might think you 'know this'. But before deciding you do 'know this' observe what you actually do on a day to day basis. If you're not doing these things then you don't really know them. Perhaps they could be things to add to your steps?

Generally, people who maintain a healthy weight year in, year out, are mainly doing these things well. Generally, people who struggle with their weight either don't do any of these very well, or they're particularly bad at one in particular. Which applies to you?

1. Eat only when you're hungry

Some people eat at pre-set meal times, whether they're hungry or not. This, like many things, is a habit. If you do this, chances are you're doing it on auto-pilot with no thought. This is an area where you should become more conscious of what you're doing. Eating when you're not hungry is keeping your fat where it is and probably making more of it for you.

Obviously, you might be eating when you're not hungry because of problems in your life - maybe you're comfort eating. That gets dealt with in the next section.

Providing you keep yourself well hydrated your body

will let you know when it needs food. When you gradually reduce your intake of food this ramps up your appetite (and increases the amount of nutritious food you eat); your hunger will accurately tell you when you need more calories.

Depending on your starting point, this may take some time to achieve, but that's okay. Many people I've worked with have not listened to their body's natural signals for so long that they don't recognise them anymore.

It's best not to let yourself get ravenously hungry if you can help it. It's just far too easy to overeat when this is your starting point. If you have a particular time of the day when you often feel like this, plan for it by having a healthy snack on you.

There's no need to get fanatical about this. For example, if you're meeting a friend for lunch and you're not quite hungry, it's fine to go ahead and eat.

2. Chew your food well

There are two very good reasons to chew your food really well. The first is that you're supposed to, that's what your teeth are for. A common cause of indigestion is that the stomach is full of food that hasn't been chewed properly. Your stomach has a lot of work to do anyway, but you really add to its work if you haven't let your mouth do its part of the job of breaking down your food.

Secondly, by chewing your food well, you also eat more slowly. Not only are you delivering food to your stomach that it can digest straightaway, you're also giving it the chance to let you know when it's full.

This also gives you the opportunity to appreciate the smell of your food. Savour every mouthful and enjoy the taste. Eating is a pleasure. Slow down and enjoy it, make the most of it.

When you eat quickly it's very easy to overshoot the mark and end up eating more than you need. You feel overfull, and possibly bloated too. Every time you feel overfull you've had more calories than you need and will be laying down body fat as a result.

3. Stop when you're satisfied
One of the biggest obstacles to this is the almost compulsive need to clear your plate. For some people it's a mortal sin to leave food.

When I was young I had to eat all my dinner if I wanted pudding (I always had room for that, even if it was a struggle to get my dinner down). At school I had to eat everything because people were starving in Africa. It can be seen as rude to leave food, especially if someone else has cooked it for you.

Maybe you have other reasons why you have to clear your plate. What are they? Whatever they are, they're probably deeply ingrained and give you a bad feeling if you leave food.

You have to get over this. For example, being fat isn't helping starving people around the world.

There are two ways to start improving in this area. Firstly, you can deliberately leave something on your plate every time you have a meal, even if it's just a small amount. The more times you do this, the more it starts to feel comfortable. This is because you're learning something new. You are consciously choosing a new behaviour, and by repetition, you're developing a new habit of stopping when you've had enough, regardless of what's on your plate.

The second way is to serve yourself a smaller portion, knowing you can go back for more if you're not satisfied by the time you've finished what's on your plate.

By doing either of these, or a combination of both, you will gradually learn the correct amount of food to put on your plate to satisfy yourself.

How do you know if you've had enough? This can take a bit practice if you commonly eat too much. You've eaten too much if you feel bloated. You want to stop before feeling particularly full. The ideal time to stop is somewhere between feeling satisfied and feeling full. You're getting there when your mouthfuls of food aren't giving you as much pleasure as previous ones – this is a signal to stop.

Some people worry that they might not eat enough and end up hungry again soon. What do you do if this happens? What do you do if you feel hungry – you eat! Even if that's two hours after a meal; if you're genuinely hungry, you eat.

This can take a bit a trial and error at first. Stick with it. Write the Hunger Scale out and have it by you when you're eating as a reminder.

I find the general advice about food portion sizes as a way of controlling calorie intake an absolute load of rubbish. This is a one size fits all (and fits with the diet mentality) approach and doesn't take into account our differences. It teaches you nothing about you. You find your own portion size by tuning in and listening to your body. Use the Hunger Scale to start with. After a while, you'll get used to how much food you need and know how much to put on your plate.

In summary:
- Eat only when you're hungry, but don't get ravenous
- Chew your food well and eat slowly – really enjoy

your food
- Stop when you're satisfied

Summary

The quality of your health and your life depends on your metabolism. The amount of body fat you have is largely a result of your metabolism.

Your muscles play a central role in your metabolism and longevity, so you need to preserve what you've got and ideally build on that by becoming more active.

There are two sides to your metabolism. Your aim is to slow down the destructive catabolic type and increase the fat burning metabolic type. You do this by eating well and looking after yourself better.

By getting your metabolism in shape you'll be rewarded not only with fat loss, but also better health. You'll be less likely to get ill, and be more likely to live longer.

Part 6 - Overcome Comfort Eating
31. Introduction

Have you ever met up with a friend for coffee, intending just to have a coffee, but on seeing the cakes and muffins, been thrown into a spin? You find yourself sat down with a big lump of cake, and you know you're going to feel guilty when you've eaten it. But you eat it anyway.

A lot of people know how to eat a lot healthier than they actually do eat i.e. more fruit and vegetables, less sugar and processed rubbish. But despite knowing this, their food choices are very different to what they know is better for them.

Comfort eating is actually a relatively new thing. Our ancestors ate when they could and they ate whatever was available. We have food available all the time and we have huge choice too. As a result, people now eat for many different reasons, and genuine physical hunger might not be at the top of your list.

The vast majority of people sometimes eat when they're not hungry, i.e. when their body doesn't need food. For some people, this turns into a seemingly uncontrollable problem that prevents them for losing their body fat.

32. Comfort Or Emotional Eating –
   What's The Cause?

Everything you eat starts with a decision. This could be because you're hungry, but in the case of the 'accidental' muffin purchase, something else was at play. Decisions about food are often preceded by a feeling or emotion. Emotions can have enormous power over your eating decisions, and they are often the complete opposite to what you want.

Comfort eating stems from a lack of a particular skill that helps a person cope with their feelings. Because these feelings aren't dealt with they are, instead, numbed with comfort food.

These skills include the ability to recognise, understand and MANAGE your emotions in a way that doesn't involve eating. The solution to comfort eating is to learn how to identify what you're feeling in that critical moment when deciding whether you need to eat, and then what to eat. Anyone can learn this. *You* can learn this if you give yourself a chance.

Learning about nutrition is really important, but if you have a problem with comfort eating, that needs to be dealt with first, otherwise this new knowledge won't get you far.

This section will teach you how to tackle this, but

reading it once will not sort your problem. The bigger the problem you have in this area, the more thought you'll need to give to it. But if you've learned to walk, talk, and drive a car, you can learn this too. Like all of these things, it takes time and practice. There is no quick fix.

Comfort Eating

People eat for many different reasons, in addition to hunger. Sometimes, there's a recurrent emotional trigger that sets you off on a regular basis. It could be boredom, stress, upset, frustration, anger, feeling low, or anxiety. Some people even overeat when they're happy.

Comfort eating isn't an all or nothing thing. To a certain extent, it effects nearly everyone. There are very few people who only ever eat in response to hunger (and I doubt they'll be reading this book). Comfort eating extends across a spectrum.

At one end you have the minority who only ever eat when they're hungry. At the other end will be the people who are totally unable to manage their emotions, except with food. These people may only rarely experience genuine physical hunger.

Only eat when hungry   Eating totally controlled by emotions

←————————→

Most people lie somewhere along this spectrum. As you learn more about your own emotions you can gradually move towards eating only when hungry. I don't think you should be aiming for this extreme, though. For example, this could be typical for someone who's relaxed around food; they eat what their body needs most of the time, but on the odd occasion, they overdo it. They could eat out with friends and feel satisfied after the main course. They may not need any more food but still fancy a bit of pudding. It's okay to do this sometimes; striving to only eat when hungry is not necessary for you to achieve your ideal weight. Perfection is not required here. Good enough will do the job nicely. Good enough is what most people of ideal weight employ.

People who successfully maintain a healthy weight, and who are relaxed and happy about eating, can enjoy sweets and puddings, but they tend to stop before they eat too much. They don't use food to soothe themselves when they feel rough during life's ups and downs. They're able to choose healthier options and not feel deprived, even if it's not their favourite thing. They tend to be in the habit (remember habits can be good) of looking beyond the meal or food choice right now, to how they're going to feel afterwards, and how it will impact their health and weight.

Successful eaters are in the habit of weighing up

the short term pleasure of what their next meal will give them against their longer-term health and weight desires. They may have done this for so long that they hardly think about it, it's just their habit now. Eight or nine times out of ten they'll choose the healthier option over the not-so-healthy one. Eight or nine times out of ten they'll stop eating when they're satisfied and not become overfull. Perfection is not at work here for the successful eater with a slim body.

The initial step towards success with your eating is understanding your emotions. First of all, you have to become aware of them. Once you raise your awareness to what's going on inside, you begin to have the choice of changing your actions from those that hurt you, to those that help you.

It's about *self-awareness*. This means tuning in to what's going on inside you rather than focusing on what's going on outside, e.g. the argument you've just had, or the stressful day at work you're having. It's about knowing yourself and recognising what's going on internally.

It's only when you become more aware of what's going on inside that you can start to *self-regulate* yourself around food. You become capable of managing your emotions in other ways separately to food.

A very simple example of this in action is recognising

you're upset because of the argument you've just had, and getting yourself out of the kitchen to do something else, knowing that the emotion you feel right now will fade if you give yourself a chance.

Most comfort eaters can predict when they'll lose control. Do any of these sound familiar?

- When I'm bored I eat almost without thinking
- After a hard day at work I deserve to have a really big meal
- When I'm stressed I can easily eat a big bar of chocolate
- After an argument with my partner or teenage kids I stuff myself
- I'm so unhappy at work, eating is my only pleasure
- It's overwhelming to think about/tackle my overeating; it's much easier to zone out the self-loathing with food that makes me feel good

What's yours?

This type of eating is in direct response to emotions. Hunger has nothing to do with it. Often the eating is done on autopilot with no thought. You are now trying to push your emotions away with food rather than dealing with them. You are trying to change your emotional state with food.

Have you ever said anything like this?

- I'm too stressed to start eating healthily right now
- I want to change my eating but I can't seem to do it, no matter how hard I try

Emotions are at the root of both of these, and until you recognise this and start dealing with it you're not going to make any progress. A lot of people who fail one attempt after another to lose weight keep repeating this mistake. They don't address their number one problem.

A lot of people ask me for food plans. While they feel good and life is going well they will happily follow these. However, as soon as a bit of stress hits them they fall off the wagon and undo all their good work by returning to old, established habits and comfort eating again.

A food plan will not help you until you deal with your problem of eating in response to your emotions.

But once you begin tackling these problems, the rest of it will fall into place and you will do very well.

Decision Time

Most people's decision making isn't always rational, even if they kid themselves it is. This is because emotions nearly always play a role to some extent. Even choosing a car has emotions wrapped up with it.

Otherwise we'd all be happy with the same thing - you wouldn't look at one car and think 'yuk', or another and think 'nice'.

Your aim is to understand how your emotions affect your decision making when it comes to food.

What emotions do you know trigger you to eat? Do you eat when you're upset, bored, stressed, angry, frustrated? Don't go any further until you've given this a bit of thought and written those initial thoughts in your notebook.

If you're a comfort eater this is what currently happens when you're triggered:

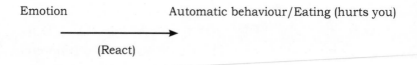

Emotion   Automatic behaviour/Eating (hurts you)

(React)

Basically, comfort eaters react to a situation without conscious thought and end up overeating, which obviously hurts them.

What you need to work towards is increasing your level of consciousness in these situations and making better decisions. It involves thinking and looks something like this:

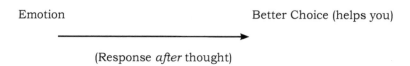

Emotion   Better Choice (helps you)

(Response *after* thought)

You'll start to recognise that a decision needs to be made, a conscious one (not an autopilot one). To do this, you have to slow down in these critical moments, enough to acknowledge that you've reached a point where a conscious decision is needed.

For example: you get home from work after a really stressful day and you head to the freezer for a tub of ice cream. This is one of the occasions where you need to wake up, out of your current default setting. You need to switch your autopilot off and change to manual. To do this, you need to pause for a moment and give yourself the opportunity to think. This is your chance to respond rather than react. Which is it going to be?

This is all about learning a new skill. When you learned to walk, you fell over loads of times. You didn't tell yourself off and nor did anyone else. Falling over is part of the learning process. Having another go is part of the learning process. Scolding yourself for failures is definitely not part of the learning process. This will massively hinder your progress, as it would a baby learning to walk.

The first part of learning this new skill is to become

conscious at these critical trigger points and switch off your autopilot. To start with, you may keep missing it. This is normal. When you know you've missed it, it's about taking a step back and thinking about it. What could you do differently next time? One of my clients put a sign on her fridge door for a while that said:

Stop! Think! Why are you eating?

Simple thought provokers like this can help train your mind to wake up from its default autopilot setting, giving you the chance to make a better choice.

Making A Decision

You have two types of decision: you can react without thought. This is likely to lead to a bad and unhealthy decision.

Or, you can respond. You can take a moment to recognise your feelings and then THINK. This gives you more chance of making a better choice.

The critical thing is taking that moment before you've reacted on autopilot. This gives you the chance to become aware. Some people take this moment by counting to ten, others have imagined pressing a pause button, or you could try a few deep breaths. Then give yourself some space to *think*.

Use this whenever you're feeling the urge to eat. Take that moment and ask yourself a few questions:

- Why do I want to eat now?
- Am I physically hungry?
- How am I feeling emotionally right now?
- Has something just happened that's triggering me to eat?

By slowing down you can become aware of what's going on inside. If you don't immediately know, you give yourself the chance to find out. If you have the urge to eat, and you're not physically hungry, you've recognised something else is prompting you to eat. What is that? Do you have a better way to deal with it?

Use this when you consider a second helping. Why do you want this?

- Are you still hungry?
- Are you going with the flow because other people are having seconds?
- It would be rude to refuse
- How are you feeling?
- Are your emotions making you want to eat more than you need?
- Are you just acting out of habit because you always have seconds?

Check how you're feeling right now. Are you feeling stressed or upset? If you are, by taking a bit of time, you give yourself a chance to respond instead of reacting. What can you do instead of eating a load of food your body doesn't need?

When you're feeling really stressed or upset, it's hard to imagine that you will feel any other way. If you're not stressed or upset right now, you know this to be the case, but when you're in the thick of it, you don't think this way. This is why, if it's your habit, it's easy to react and soothe yourself with food. Taking that moment out is essential.

People who manage their emotions well and who don't make a bee-line for the fridge when they're upset, do something different. They know this feeling will lessen, given a bit of time. They'll say things to themselves like:

- This feeling will pass
- I've been here before and got through it
- This is horrible, but I can handle it

They might do something like a simple breathing exercise to get a grip of themselves. They might go out for a walk to clear their head, or call a friend and have a chat. They could put music on that they know makes them feel good. They might even clean their kitchen cupboards!

These things serve as a distraction while the intensity of the emotion subsides. As it lessens you can cope with it without food. You have to switch off your autopilot for this to start working. You have to become conscious and think.

Taking Control

Most people try to tackle their weight problem by going on a diet. Even if you aren't a comfort eater, going on a diet is a recipe for disaster. But most people who are overweight have some degree of emotions directing their eating. Diets don't fix this problem, which is another reason they fail. As a comfort eater, you know this, but until now you haven't had an alternative.

Your moment of power is when you pause to think. This will take a little while to get into the habit. At first, you'll miss it more than you hit it. This is normal. It's only by practice and thought that you will get better. Any time you beat yourself up about getting it wrong, take a step back.

Criticising yourself puts your focus on what you did wrong. This makes you more likely to repeat the same mistake again. It's much better to accept you've made a mistake then think about how you can do better next time. Even more effective is to imagine yourself doing it right next time. This helps to program your mind for a better outcome.

You're aiming to make a conscious decision each time you eat. Before eating, take a moment to think; press the pause button. This gives you the chance to recognise how you're feeling. The more you do this (and record what you notice in your notebook), the more you will understand how your emotions direct not only your food choices, but how much you eat too.

If you truly have to eat you could choose a granola bar or flapjack instead of a massive bag of crisps or entire tub of ice cream. It's about giving yourself the space to make a conscious choice rather than reacting and being at the mercy of your emotions.

One client of mine had a really difficult relationship with her ex-husband. They were still in regular contact because of their son. She'd done one diet after another over the years in the attempt to shed four stone. Instead, she gradually got fatter. Like many comfort eaters, she had little trouble eating healthily when life went smoothly, but when she got stressed that would go out of the window. Interaction with her ex was a common trigger. Here's an extract from an email she sent me:

*I have to speak with Mike at least twice a month and I nearly always feel upset and angry after. He's such an unreasonable *******! I either shake with anger or I'm in tears even before the conversation is over. I noticed that this always triggered a big blow out. I'd eat* *anything I could get my hands on. It would completely derail me from my healthy eating plan. Because I felt like I'd completely blown it, I would carry on eating cakes, biscuits, chocolate, and loads of sweet stuff, for a few days. I just wouldn't care; I'd blown it after all, what was the point? I stopped exercising too. Then I'd get a grip a few days later but always feel really guilty and stupid.*

I already knew that a conversation with Mike would most likely trigger a binge. It wasn't as if this eating binge came out of the blue. It was predictable. I sat down and thought about how I could handle it better next time. I planned to go out of the house, crying or not, and walk for half an hour.

The next time Mike phoned I forgot all about this plan until I'd eaten all the ice cream in the fridge, and my son's sweets. I felt ashamed and useless. But then I remembered not to beat myself up and instead think about it. I had 'fallen over' and needed to get back up.

The next time Mike tried his (bad) magic on me I remembered to leave the house immediately I got off the phone. I remembered because I left a post-it note by the phone, which I stuck over the keypad as soon as I knew it was him. When I slammed the phone down I noticed the note, grabbed my keys and slammed the front door on my way out.

As I stomped around the block my anger and upset lessened. By the time I got home, I felt calm and in control again, and I didn't need to eat. I felt very emotional, in a good way - almost teary. I realised then that I could take control back.

This is a great example of thought in action. She knew that this situation prompted her to overeat, so planned for it. She decided ahead of time what her distraction technique would be. It didn't work the first time; she reacted on autopilot and ate loads of food instead. But she tweaked her plan, didn't give up, or think she was useless. She recognised that this was a learning process that would take time and involve a few mistakes along the way. The post-it note served as a great thought provoker. It knocked her into 'manual mode' rather than sailing off on autopilot. Her new plan was there in front of her: Go for a walk. Do not pass fridge. Do not collect ice cream!

She had another upsetting phone call. She felt horrible after this. It's okay to feel horrible for a short period of time, it won't kill you. A half an hour walk was enough for this woman to feel in control again.

Her ex-husband wasn't the only thing that upset her. The more she practised her new choice of behaviour after interacting with her ex, the more she noticed other times she felt upset. More and more she took a moment in these situations, consciously thinking about her decision to eat or not. Did she really need some food or did she need to take time out and calm down instead?

Once you get into the habit of recognising how you feel and pause to think, you're able to make the choice to manage your feelings in other ways than eating. What way could you manage your emotional calls to eat better? Would doing something physical suit you, i.e. going for a walk, cleaning, or just generally tidying something up? Maybe doing something to connect with someone would be better for you - you could have a chat with someone on the phone, write an email, pop in to see an elderly neighbour. Perhaps doing something to use your mind is more your thing, such as writing a list of everything you need to do for your upcoming holiday, or just a shopping list.

It's good to think ahead, because if you leave it until the heat of the moment, you're bound to go for the far easier option and just eat. When you catch yourself and give yourself the option of a better decision, you don't want to be left floundering and not knowing what to do instead. Plan ahead. If you know you eat out of boredom, what can you do to relieve your boredom? What's going to work well for you? Have a Plan B up your sleeve ready for the next time you recognise boredom rearing its head. Give yourself a fighting chance.

When a friend of mine started working from home he also started putting on weight. This was because he was bored. When he'd been bored at work he'd have a quick chat with work colleagues, he didn't think about eating. After a quick chat he would be back to his work again. With no one to talk with at home he wandered into the kitchen and ate things instead.

His solution was to recognise his boredom and, instead of eating, go out for a quick walk with the dog. This served as a quick break, then he felt refreshed and ready to work again, without eating half a packet of biscuits.

Recognising Self Sabotage

While you've been reading this section have you been saying to yourself anything like this?
- This won't work for me
- I'll try it when I get back from my holiday, there's no point before
- I've got too much on right now to try this, maybe later

Recognise this for what it is - you are sabotaging yourself and shooting yourself in your foot before you even start. You can decide right now not to sabotage yourself and just get on with it. Or, you can skim over this without giving it much thought. It's your choice.

Just getting ready is the start of the process. You can think about what you've read. How does this translate into your life? What can you do for yourself in this regard? You should have plenty of thoughts, and even plans, to write in your notebook.

This is a big area that's going to require *more* thought than action. You crystallise your thoughts by putting them down on paper and reviewing them. If you just passively read this section without thinking and planning, you'll not overcome your problems with comfort and emotional eating. The action bit is actually a very small part of this, most of it needs to take place inside your head.

In Summary

The nuts and bolts of this seem quite easy when written down. But any new skill takes time and practice. If you think you can learn a new a skill by missing the time and practice bit out you're wrong. Here are the steps towards learning something new.

1. Recognise how your emotions influence your eating choices
2. Take a moment when these emotions rear their head
3. Accept that it's okay to feel these emotions, rather than immediately reacting to them and numbing them with food

4. Give yourself time to respond; give yourself chance to make a conscious decision, rather than revert back to your current default setting

5. Choose to do something different. Choose to help yourself

33. Dealing With Comfort Eating

You've got some insight now as to why you lose control around food. Next, you need some tools to deal with this.

A shortened version of the example I gave:

- Before - I overate because I got angry and upset with my ex
- After - I still got stressed and upset with my ex and wanted to eat, so I went for a walk to calm down instead, knowing this feeling would pass if I just gave it chance
- Result - I feel in control and have taken a positive step towards being healthier

This is all about noticing and recognising the feelings inside. You need to look inside and see what it is you're feeling in these moments that precede eating unnecessarily. What is it for you? Is it stress, upset, anger, boredom? Maybe you can't put your finger on it exactly, but it's not good.

Once you noticed you've hit a danger point - you

recognise the feeling - it's time to take a moment and make a conscious decision about what you're going to do. Are you going to give in to your feelings and eat (and hurt yourself), or are you going to choose something different that will take you in the direction you want to go? It's your choice, you do have one.

Everyone is on autopilot at times, whether they're a comfort eater or not. You'll have driven somewhere, and when you got there, not remembered much about the journey. That's because it was a journey you're used to doing and you switched over to autopilot. Someone stepping out in front of you would soon have you back in the moment and concentrating. At this point, you become aware. You have to respond to this situation.

It's not only comfort eaters who get to the end of a packet of crisps and think 'where did they go?' You can't remember eating them all because you switched off and mindlessly munched your way through them. Maybe you were reading a book or watching TV at the same time.

As mentioned previously, you're aiming to be conscious when you eat and to be aware of each mouthful. It's being in the moment; it's being tuned in to what's going on right now. But for you, the comfort eater, it's also vital to 'be here' while deciding if and what to eat too. You might need some kind of thought provoker at the beginning while you're getting the hang of it.

Being in the moment means focusing on the task in hand. You either have your mind focused on the decision you're about to make (rather than being on autopilot), or you are enjoying your food. You're not thinking or worrying about past or future events. You're totally focused on what you are doing now, in the here and now.

Wanting To Eat Versus Needing To Eat

Needing to eat, because your body is hungry for food, is all about listening to and recognising your internal cues. Where are you on the hunger scale? Are you actually hungry? Do you even need to eat right now?

The Hunger Scale
1 – Feeling faint
2 – Absolutely ravenous
3 – Quite hungry
4 – Peckish
5 – Neutral
6 – Satisfied
7 – Full
8 – Over full
9 – Stuffed and bloated
10 – So full you could vomit
Eat when you notice yourself at 3 or 4

When you're not in tune with your body it's easy to confuse emotional hunger with physical hunger. Until you become tuned into your body these two can feel similar. However, there are differences. Emotional hunger tends to be sudden and urgent; it needs to be satisfied now! Physical hunger builds up gradually, it doesn't come out of nowhere.

When you have a sudden or desperate craving for food, it's time to tune into yourself to find out what's going on inside, before burying those feelings with food.

Genuine physical hunger is gradual. You may notice things like a gentle rumbling or a little griping. When you don't satisfy this it gradually builds, and given time, you'll become ravenous and even feel faint.

You may eat in response to negative emotions, but how much do you react to external cues? We're manipulated left, right and centre at the supermarket. If you don't go in with a pre-planned list, and stick to it, you've pretty much had it. As soon as you walk in you'll be faced with a display of tempting cakes and pastries that smell wonderful and are probably pretty cheap. They're carefully placed for the impulse buyer. Do you fall for this?

If you manage to get past that, do you resist all the treats at the checkout? How often do you see pieces of fruit at the checkout? Think about it. This is all planned to part you from your money, fuel your addiction, make you come back for more, make you put more weight on, and destroy your health.

How many times have you popped into a supermarket with the intention of buying just a few bits but come out with all sorts? As far as the advertising in the supermarket is concerned, you've been manipulated nicely and have responded perfectly.

Don't go food shopping when you're hungry, and always have a list!
Have you gone into your kitchen cupboard, not thinking about crisps, but on seeing them, suddenly wanting them? How about walking through a shopping centre? You're not thinking about eating, but on seeing a little stall selling biscuits or hot dogs, you suddenly want to eat.

Most of us react to external cues to some extent. A lot of people will deny they do, because they don't even realise they're doing so. You need to raise your level of awareness and identify these. This easy exercise will take you through the thought processes involved.

- Before eating anything train yourself to THINK
- Do you 'need' to eat? Where are you on the hunger scale - are you physically hungry?
- Do you just want to eat? Where are you on a scale

of 1-10 (with 1 being a low level and 10 being a
high level of 'want' to eat this food)
- Compare these scores
- If your 'want' is higher than your 'need' it's time to
take a moment and think, because your emotions
and/or you are being overly influenced by external
cues at play

An example of this in practice could be that you've
just been offered a lump of chocolate cake. Your 'want'
is scoring at a 9 - you really want this! However, your
'need' scores really low because you're not hungry.
There are two ways to play this:
1. You might think: 'what the heck, you only live
   once!' and eat the cake. This is fine 1-2 times out
   of 10, and slim people do this. However, if you
   do this all the time, or even 8-9 times out of 10,
   you've got a problem.
2. You accept you want the cake, but you take a
   moment to think about what you might want even
   more than that. What's your goal? Imagine it for a
   few seconds. Do you really want this cake today?
   It's not that you can never have chocolate cake -
   it's not forbidden. You're not on a diet, after all.

This might seem like a lot to do, but when you're
used to it, it will become automatic and you'll be able
to make your decision in seconds. This is what a
successful eater will do on autopilot, almost without
thought. What you practice gradually becomes your

default automatic behaviour and it becomes easy.

Doing this might feel a bit weird, or even wrong at first. Fold your arms. Now fold them the other way. That feels a bit weird, doesn't it? But it's not wrong; it's just different, something you're not used to.

Trying something new, even if it feels wrong, requires you to open your mind. There is more than one way to fold your arms! When your mind is open you're prepared to try something new to get something new, i.e. your slim and healthy body. When your mind is closed you keep doing the same things but expect a different result. According to Einstein, this is insanity (and therefore doesn't work). These are examples of people doing the same things and expecting a different result to the last time they did it:

- Repeatedly dieting (even if they're different diets)
- Repeatedly trying to use willpower to succeed

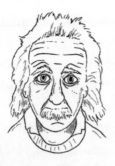

'Insanity is doing the same thing over and over again and expecting different results'

- Albert Einstein

If you choose to keep your mind closed, because all this feels too weird, you'll remain stuck with your current habits. You'll revert back to your old, established habits, and keep repeating the same mistakes (doing the same things and expecting a different result) - and stay fat.

You have to do different things to
get something different!

This is a closed mind in action: 'I was stressed and I needed crisps, so I had them'. End of story.

This is an open mind in action: 'I recognised and accepted that I felt stressed in that moment. I felt the urge to eat but I remembered, just in time, that the intensity of this feeling would pass. I chatted with friends on Facebook to distract myself while the stress and urge to eat settled.'

Which will you choose?

Accepting Your Feelings Rather Than Ignoring Them

Before you can start managing your emotions without food, you need to start understanding what your hot buttons are. How do specific things make you feel? Do you have problem times during the day?

Most people, if they sat and THOUGHT about it, could predict their difficult times just like a weather man predicts the weather. You can prepare for it. If you know it's going to rain you can take a coat with you. This won't work every single time - you're bound to get caught out now and then, but most of the time you'll be prepared. And it's most of the time that counts. Getting it right all of the time is not necessary.

When are you likely to fall down?

When you do fall down and get it wrong, do you feel guilty? How does this help you? It doesn't help in any way at all so you must get rid of it. Guilt just makes you feel bad, knocks your self-esteem, and puts your focus exactly where you don't want it (making it more likely that you'll repeat the same mistake again). How productive would it be to make a child feel bad for falling off their bike when they're learning to ride it?

Your goal of fat loss is really important, but the process may not be easy. ACCEPT that the whole thing gets easier because you can be gentler and encouraging with yourself.

A lot of people have a habit of overeating at night. They can be 'good' all day and then blow it in the evening. If this is you, you know this is likely to happen, so you can predict this. Therefore, you can PREPARE your plan of action in advance, rather than waiting for it to keep happening (like Groundhog Day). Knowing yourself gives you power (providing you act on that knowledge).

Here's an example of how one of my clients tackled this:

I used to skip breakfast and not eat much during the day at work. Work is very stressful and I would get home feeling really hungry and like I deserved to eat a lot, because I'd been so busy all day. I would eat a huge amount in the evening and go to bed completely bloated nearly every night.

I couldn't stomach breakfast at first (probably because I'd eaten so much the night before), but I started taking healthy snacks and a packed lunch to work. I wasn't starving when I got home but I still wanted to eat a lot because of the stress.

I would get in and, while drinking a big glass of water, sit down with my notebook and read my goal, and remind myself what I wanted to achieve. This would get me in a better frame of mind. Because I'd already planned what to eat (I make a food plan at the weekend and plan my shopping around it) everything was there to make a healthy meal.

I would not watch the TV until I finished eating; this would stop me mindlessly eating and eating.

I still enjoyed some chocolate after my food but would break off a few squares onto a plate and eat only them. This stopped me eating a whole bar every night.

Gradually, I developed an appetite in the morning, and so started to have breakfast. This was something new for me, and I realised it was because I was no longer overeating at night.

A lot of thought went into this, followed by a lot of practice. I have no doubt this person had a few evenings where it all went wrong and she overate. You've just got to start again tomorrow when this happens, without beating yourself up!

Maybe you have a challenging relationship with someone close to you – your partner or your children. You know that difficult interactions with them press your buttons and cause you to eat. You may react like usual (closed mind if you continue like this) and say 'I've had enough! Eating is the only thing that will help me feel better. I can't help it!' Or you can take a moment to think and RESPOND in your new, planned-in-advance way (because you've opened your mind to something new), and say, 'I'm stressed and I don't like feeling like this. Instead of running to the fridge, I'm going to run myself a hot bath and have a nice soak while I settle down.'

What do you intend to do the next time your 'button' is pressed? Preparation is key here. Write this down in your notebook.

What's the purpose of putting a child on the naughty

step? It's to give them time out to cool down. You're expecting them to sit with their feelings, think things through and then behave better or, at least, differently. By giving yourself a bit of time out when your button is pressed, you're doing the same thing. It involves you sitting with your feelings for a while, instead of stuffing them down with food.

Perhaps you've just got into the habit of overeating. This behaviour might be automatic for you because you've done it for so long. Sitting with the hunger scale next to you and asking yourself where you are on it throughout the meal can help you tune into your body's signals. In time, you won't need the scale, you'll just know.

It can be challenging to change established habits, because you've got to notice them first. You've got to catch yourself and interrupt the autopilot. In the beginning, you'll miss this more often than not - that's normal.

On average, it takes 66 days to cement a new habit. This is why you can't rush these things. It's only by taking the time needed that you'll ultimately succeed. You have to be patient with yourself.

Writing things in your notebook is really important while you're going through this process. It focuses your mind, helps you think clearly and helps you make better plans for change. Those who do this, and who regularly write in their notebooks, will do better. It means you're giving things thought. If you feel resistance to this, you're likely to sabotage yourself. This sabotage could be dressed up as having 'no time' or having trouble writing anything because it might not be 'right'. This is the time to open your mind and get on with it!

Doing Something Different

Eating is often an ingrained response to a feeling, and it takes time to learn something new, just like when you learned to drive. And just like when you learned to drive, you're going to have little setbacks.

Repetition is the key to learning anything new. You're aiming to tune into your feelings before you eat. By doing this, you'll give yourself the chance to make better decisions. Eventually, your better decisions will become your new, ingrained habits.

It's not uncommon to eat well for a while then suddenly mindlessly eat a load of chocolate, or whatever your comfort food is. In these situations it's good to remind yourself that this is a process. When you notice what you're doing, or what you've done, it's time to THINK. It's not time to think 'what the hell, I may as well go on a huge binge now'.

It's helpful to change the way you talk to yourself. For example, when you say something like 'I can't have chocolate cake', you're speaking from a diet mentality. Compare that to saying this: 'I choose not to have chocolate cake right now'. Saying it like this makes it a personal choice rather than an old, ingrained diet habit telling you what to do. No one likes being told what to do, even by themselves. A lot of people naturally do the opposite to what they're told. The words you use to talk to yourself matter.

Eating out often causes people problems. This is definitely a time to remain conscious and tuned in to yourself. The good thing about eating out is that it's usually planned in advance. This gives you time to think things through and to prepare. Hold the hunger scale in the front of your mind when ordering, and also when deciding whether to have pudding or not. Rather than getting swept along with old habits, or with what everyone else is doing, take time to think and tune in to what's going on inside – do this before choosing.

If you're tempted with seconds or pudding and you're already quite full, imagine yourself two hours later. How are you going to enjoy feeling stuffed and bloated, knowing you could have stopped eating instead and felt okay? This is something successful eaters do on autopilot. If you've ordered too much food and don't want to waste it, get it put into a doggie bag and take it home.

Some people say that they have a loud voice inside their head that they can't say no to. It says things like:

- I want cake
- I want crisps
- I want a doughnut
- I want seconds

This voice gets more insistent if it's ignored.

Rather than trying to ignore it, which doesn't usually work, break this down and THINK. Think about this in terms of 'now' versus 'later'. With the 'now' you get a small payoff by indulging this impulsive desire to eat. The payoff is usually very short-lived, because as soon as you've eaten it, you feel regret and guilt. With the 'later' you know you're heading towards your goal of fat loss and that you're going to spare yourself the regret and guilt.

I always have pudding, or at least I used to. Even if I was bloated after my meal I would always stuff a pudding down, this is just what I did. I never really thought about it.

I realised this wasn't helping me and I addressed this problem first. At the end of my main meal I would go inside and imagine how fat and bloated I would feel

*after having a pudding too. Not good! Then I would
imagine feeling okay in half an hour instead, because I
didn't have pudding. I would also imagine myself slim
and feeling good in the future.*

*Most of the time this was enough and the urge to have
pudding went away. I felt really good not having the
pudding! Sometimes, I would still have pudding, if
I wasn't really full already. I feels good having the
choice.*

However, there could be something else going on here.
Where do you think your blood sugar is? What were
you eating earlier – was it good, slow-release food, or
was it refined carbs? Has it been a long time since you
ate; have you got too hungry? In this situation, your
'eat signal' is especially strong for unhealthy foods
and the 'now' reward becomes bigger than your 'later'
reward.

Don't make this harder on yourself than it needs to
be. Eat regularly, eat well, keep your blood sugar
stable and avoid this.

34. Obstacles To Overcome Comfort Eating

What I've written before might sound all very well,
but chances are, you'll have something going on that
may prevent you putting this into practice. There are
a number of reasons you may struggle, and the first

step towards dealing with them is recognising them. You need to bring them up to the surface and look at them. What follows are a few pitfalls that may hinder your progress when overcoming your comfort eating. It may be that more than one of these will be relevant to you.

Dieting

A deeply ingrained diet mentality is perhaps one of the most common reasons people struggle to get on top of their comfort eating problem. I've said so much about the harm and dangers of dieting already that, at the very least, it should have prompted a fair bit of thought.

When you diet, decisions about what you eat are based on rules given by the diet. It takes absolutely no account of how you feel. Diets seem to completely ignore the fact that a person's feelings will nearly always win out in the end. But you tend to blame yourself when it/you fails, rather than the stupid diet. The more times this happens, the bigger a failure you feel. You get to the point where you think nothing will work for you. This simply isn't true, you just need to work in harmony with your body AND your feelings. Diets can't do this for you.

Serial dieters tend to have significant psychological struggles around food. This shows itself as:

- Feeling afraid to eat
- Worrying about what you just ate, and maybe guilt too
- Worrying about what you plan to eat
- Counting calories and/or fat content
- Worrying about being hungry
- A minor setback triggering a binge for the rest of the day: 'I've blown it, I might as well make the most of it.'

All these things make you feel bad, and increase your likelihood of comfort eating to make yourself feel better. Comfort eating can give you temporary relief from the horrible 'diet mood'.

Dieting leads to distorted eating, because you're no longer listening to the messages from your body. You might be skipping meals one day then binge-eating another. You end up either resisting your hunger, or caving in and going completely overboard. There's no tuning into yourself and becoming aware of how you're feeling; no consideration towards making your own conscious decisions.

Healthy eating is not based on rigid rules. It's flexible and pleasurable. When you learn to manage your emotions and start making logical decisions about your eating:

- *You* decide what to eat
- *You* decide when to eat

- *You* decide how much to eat
- *You* respond to cravings by THINKING first

You must ditch the diet if you want to become healthy and slim.

Pleasure-seeking

This one takes some unpicking for most people, and involves some thinking. Whilst eating should always be pleasurable, you need to watch out for a few things.

Feel-good neurotransmitters are released in the brain when you eat sugary and refined food. This gives you a short-term hit and lines you up nicely to crave the same sort of food again, very soon. If you find yourself craving this sort of food you need to pause and think why. Is it just an old habit rearing its head because you used to eat a lot of this kind of junk? Have you recently had this kind of food and the come-down is driving your appetite for more?

It's okay to want food that gives you pleasure, but it's important to take that extra step and look at what's underneath it. Are you stressed, bored, unhappy? Give your mind some space to see what's going on, then you'll be able to make an 'informed' decision, rather than just reacting in your old way. If you identify that you feel bored, and that's triggering your pleasure-seeking receptors, what will you do instead? Have you got your plan written down in your notebook? You should literally be writing yourself a manual here of how to conquer all these problems.

As you get better at this you will sometimes choose to indulge. But you'll have done that after conscious thought. Other times, you'll pass. This takes time, but with practice, you'll get there.

You have to give yourself a chance to think when it comes to mastering impulsive eating. When you feel that impulse to eat, think about the gains you'll make, by either not eating or choosing something healthier (it doesn't have to be a perfect choice). What are your goals, right from the beginning of the book? What's it going to be like fitting into your clothes and looking good? Because it's only natural to be more swayed by short-term benefits, you could think about these things before making your decision too:

- In five minutes time I won't feel any guilt
- I won't feel full and bloated, I'll just feel nice
- I'll feel really pleased with myself for being in control

The other useful thing to do in the 'impulsive eating situation' is to check out what your expectations are about this impulsive eat. When you feel unhappy, bored, or stressed, you impulsively eat comfort food, because in that moment, you believe it makes you feel better. Expectations are very powerful at pushing you into action, and you can keep eating and eating in the hope of eventually feeling better.

THINK about how you will feel. You might think 'this chocolate will help me feel better', and this is probably your old habitual program running. Is it really going to make you feel better? For how long? A person who thinks, rather than reacting, will change this thought into something like this 'I only think this chocolate will help, and if it does, it will only be for a few minutes, then I'll feel guilty, on top of all this stress'. THINK, and do something different.

Everyone craves pleasurable foods sometimes, even slim people. This is a fact of life in today's world. So don't expect to be totally free of this, it's unlikely to happen. This is why you have to learn how to manage it. When you learn this, sometimes you indulge, sometimes you don't, because you're focused on the future benefits.

When all this starts falling into place, and you can fully enjoy food again, you can feel better about eating less. Start doing these things to really appreciate the food you're eating:
- Always sit down and focus on what's on your plate
- Look at your food and appreciate it
- Enjoy the smells coming from your food
- Savour the taste of each mouthful

- Appreciate the texture as you chew
- Absolutely savour each and every mouthful

Eating is a pleasure, and you get to do it at least three times a day. Increase your enjoyment by 'being there' in the moment and savouring it. Don't waste this enjoyment by mindlessly shoving it all in.

Eating With Other People

I'll start this section with a blog entry I wrote in 2014.

How aware are you, regarding how other people influence your eating decisions, especially in social settings?

If you intend to make a lifestyle change that gets you healthier, like improving your eating, people will either help you or hinder you.

People Who Help You
These people will probably have a healthy and relaxed relationship with food themselves. People like this generally make their own decisions about the food they eat and they can easily say 'no' when they don't want any more.

For example, they might be at a friend's for dinner and offered a slice of home-made cake for pudding. They're really full, so they say something like 'I'm full, so no

thanks, I'll take my slice home and have it tomorrow'.
They can say this with confidence and politeness and
not offend their friend.

People like this help you for two reasons. Firstly, they
demonstrate how to stop when you've had enough and
how to make a confident decision regardless of what
others are doing. Secondly, they're not concerned with
your choice - your choice is your choice – they don't try
to persuade you one way or another.

People Who Don't Help You

Unfortunately, there are many more of these about, and
there is often nothing deliberate behind this hindrance.
But it's really important to become aware of them,
so you can prevent this often unintentional sabotage
to your good intentions. It's especially important to
become aware of this if you live with someone who
does this to you.

Hinderers encourage you to eat or drink more than
you would if you were left to your own devices. They
might say things like 'oh, go on, have a pudding. I'll
feel greedy if it's just me having one', or 'you're no fun
since you started getting healthy', or 'have another
drink'.

The intention might be good here, BUT it isn't helping
you, therefore it's harming you.

What To Do

Notice the helpers in your life and study how they are around food. What can you learn from them that you can start doing?

Set your own boundaries around food, be ready to stand your ground and stick to your guns. If you find it hard to say 'no, thank you' start practising! If you really want to lose some weight it's time to stop going with the flow and dancing to someone else's tune.

Lastly, do you help or hinder the people in your life, regarding their choices around food? When you start helping and encouraging others, you help yourself too.

The more you're swayed by other people, and social cues, the more you're likely to eat. When you're eating with others do you:

- Follow the crowd, i.e. wait and see what other people order first?
- Fall victim to 'group eat'?
- Copy what others do, instead of making up your own mind?

Start becoming aware of how other people influence you.

When you're eating with others take a moment before ordering and THINK. What's going on outside? What are other people doing or saying? More importantly, what's going on inside? Where are you on the hunger scale? Where are you regarding need and wanting food?

You might be someone who wants to please. If you have a strong desire to please others you're more likely to overeat in company. Perhaps you've eaten a pudding, or said yes to an extra helping, just to please. Maybe you recognised you didn't really want it, but had it anyway, for fear of offending.

If this is you – become aware of it. Then you'll have a better chance of taking a moment and tuning into yourself. Do you really want the extra food? Are you hungry? Are you tempted to say yes, just to please? How is this behaviour helping you? For example, you might be out with your partner and they're hungrier than you. They say 'let's have dessert!' On autopilot, you just say yes, without thinking. If you give yourself a chance to think, you can tune into how you're feeling. Do you really want a pudding? If yes, go for it. If no, act accordingly.

When you know you're going to be eating socially, think about it beforehand. How do you want to be?

I would be awful for completely overeating at any buffet style meal. It was silly, but a small part of me would worry that if I didn't get in first and pile my plate high there wouldn't be anything left for me. I would be scared of going hungry. It was almost like a competitive thing – how much could I get on my plate; how quickly could I eat it so I could go back for more?

Because of the changes I had made at home I got used to how much food I needed on my plate to satisfy my hunger. During buffets I still feel that stressful feeling coming before I get to the food, but I know that it's an old habit. I also know that it will be there until I have my new habit nailed down.

I am now choosing to do something different. I put enough food on my plate to satisfy me (well, maybe a little more, just in case). The rest of the evening is more enjoyable as I'm not bloated. I also don't have to carry the guilt of eating too much. If that fear of not having had enough to eat comes up, and the food has all gone so I can't get any more, I calm myself down. The worst case scenario here is I can eat something when I get home.

A new relationship is often a time when people put on a load of weight. Usually, you get a convergence of eating behaviours, commonly in line with the person who's more dominant with regards to this particular habit. One, or both, of you will increase or decrease weight. Often, it's weight gain.

You eat together. It's pleasurable to do this, it helps with bonding. Later, you fall into the habit of eating the same thing because it's easier.

If you find yourself in the situation where you want to change but your partner doesn't, the worst thing you can do is try and force your partner to change. This is not likely to work and will only create arguments. You have to take charge of what you eat and not try and change your partner. If this means eating different things, so be it. You have to decide what you want, and what's important to you. Do you want to stay overweight and worry about your health for an easy life? Or are you going to take the bull by the horns this time and do something about it?

The best thing to do with a resistant partner is to go there first yourself. Don't tell them what to do, just do what you want to do. If you are calm, in control and determined, your partner may see the changes in you and gradually come round to making some changes themself. But it's is their choice.

I'd been putting off losing weight for years, using my husband as an excuse, because he wasn't interested in doing it either. I guess I didn't want to do it on my own, and also thought preparing a different meal for me would be too much effort.

When I got diagnosed with diabetes (due to my weight) I knew I had to do something. It turned out to be a lot easier than I thought. My husband didn't have to drink lots of water for me to start doing it. He didn't have to have large portions of steamed vegetables and less rice or fewer potatoes on his plate for me to start doing that either.

He wasn't supportive at the beginning but he came round. Once we both accepted we were doing different things, it was okay. He continues to eat what he wants. I hope he will change too, but that's up to him.

If you're getting no support at home you can get involved with my membership club where you will get weekly support.

Stress

A lot of people think 'the way they are' is just 'the way they are', and they can't change that. You might think you don't handle stress well, because that's 'the way you are'. If you know this to be true then it will be, because your mind is closed to the possibility of change. And for you, it's just 'the way you are', so there's no point trying to change. End of story.

However, when you accept that stress is something you can *learn* to deal with better, you open your mind to the possibility you can master this problem and enjoy your life more. You can learn how to be better at anything you want with the right information, but it starts with *knowing* it's possible. And since other

people have learned how to cope with stress, so can
you.

If your current ability to handle stress is a bit on the
low side, you'll brood and obsess over things, rather
than letting them go. You can become emotionally and
physically frazzled by stress. If, instead of dealing with
your stress, you try and wait it out, you're probably
decreasing the quality of your life and increasing your
waistline in the process.

You might have put off making changes to your life
and health because of current stressful situations.
'I'll lose weight after my divorce'; 'I'll get healthier
when I get past this work deadline'; 'when the kids go
back to school I'll make a start'. Stress is constantly
ebbing and flowing in your life – this is normal and
it happens to everyone. What's important is how you
deal with it. Are you going to continue using stress as
a reason not to get yourself sorted out? It is possible
to deal with stress without eating; you can lose
weight while life's normal stresses go up and down in
your life. It's all about doing something different and
learning a different way.

People who handle their stress well can talk
themselves down from it, and don't resort to eating to
push their feelings away. Their self-talk is different;
they talk themselves down by saying things like
'This is horrible but I can handle it'. They might call

a friend for a chat or go out for a walk to clear their head. Or they might just let it go, if it's something they can't do anything about.

If you're a 'stress eater' you're more likely to revert to an automatic, ingrained behaviour when your stress buttons have been hit. When you're stressed you can still make a solid decision, but it requires THOUGHT, not free-wheeling on autopilot. When you notice you're feeling stressed (noticing is obviously a critical step) you have to give yourself space to THINK. It is only when you do this that you give yourself a chance to make a better decision. You give yourself the opportunity to focus beyond what is happening at that moment.

One of my clients had a big problem with this. She said, 'Everything I know about healthy eating goes right out the window when I'm feeling stressed!' Yes, this does feel hard at first, but make it easier on yourself by having a plan for the next time stress hits you, and those 'I must eat now' moments come up.

What she did was say to herself (out loud, if on her own) 'STOP!' when she noticed the 'I must eat now, because I'm stressed' feelings. Her intention was to give herself some mental space to THINK. If she was particularly wound up she'd choose one of these two easy ways to calm down.

1. Calming breathing exercise – Take a slow, deep breath in, to the count of three. Feel your lungs fill all the way down to the bottom. Slowly let your breath out to a count of six. Feel your lungs empty completely. While doing this, focus entirely on your breath going in and out. Keep doing this until you feel more in control.

2. Calming relaxation exercise – It's impossible to feel stressed when the muscles in your body are relaxed. Mind and body are linked. Start with your face and let all the tension drop out of it; feel your facial muscles relax. Then move your focus to your shoulders and arms. Let your shoulders drop a little and feel your arms go loose. Feel your torso relax, and then your legs, all the way down to your toes. The upper part of your body might have started to tense up again by this point; if so, start again. Keep focusing on relaxing your muscles.

Doing either one of these will bring your stress down a good few notches. This gives you the opportunity to THINK about what you want to do, rather than reacting out of habit.

Is this something you can just let go? This involves accepting something as it is, and not trying to change it.

Is it time to put your Plan B into action? What have you thought about **before**, for these situations? What are you going to do instead of eating?

You've stopped your automatic behaviour, you've calmed yourself down, you've given yourself space to THINK, and you have your plan that you created before this moment. You're in the ideal position to choose something else. You've given yourself choice, something you may have felt was missing before. Are you going to choose in a way that helps you, or which continues to harm you? It is now entirely your choice.

It's also important to do the general things that help you manage your stress:

- Get enough sleep
- Eat healthy foods
- Decrease things that stress your body – alcohol, caffeine, nicotine
- Get some regular exercise

Trauma

This is perhaps the most difficult of all obstacles to overcome, and reading a book might not be enough for you to deal with this. I'm writing about it briefly for entirety, but if you have some big trauma in your past you may need some therapy to get past it.

Two people could be involved in the same car accident. One of them manages to get back in the car and drive again very soon after. The other suffers

post-traumatic stress disorder, and experience
flashbacks, nightmares, and they're unable to get
back into a car.

Challenging experiences can completely skew your
emotions, leading to ongoing problems, including
overeating as a way to push such feelings away. These
experiences can be varied: a divorce, a bereavement,
rape or sexual abuse, bullying, illness, a bad accident,
etc. Things like this can shatter your sense of control
and security.

People are different in the way they deal with horrible
things. Most people come to a point of closure, after
going through the normal stages of shock, anger, and
sadness. Others find no resolution and old problems
can be buried under many pounds of excess weight.

Overeating can develop as a way to cope with very
painful feelings caused by a traumatic event. Feelings
are pushed away with food. Making the connection
with overeating and past traumatic experience isn't
always easy, especially if it happened a long time ago.

Sharing things with a friend or counsellor may help
the healing process. You might need specialised
therapy; if you think you do, take the first step.

You can go and see your doctor, have an initial
chat, and get referred. Working in the NHS, I know

specialised psychological treatment is a bit patchy, and some areas are better served than others. You also may have to wait for your therapy, but it's still worth checking out.

Do you know anyone who has had therapy? Can they recommend a good therapist? You could look online and find someone there. When you find one that looks suitable, read the testimonials from previous clients. I would go a step further and ask if there are any who would talk with you, so you can get a good feel if this therapist will be right for you.

35. Summary

Comfort and emotional eating are things you can overcome. It may not be easy, but you can do it. It may take you longer than you would like, but if you keep at it, _you can do it_.

Most of the work is done in your head; you have to think your way out of comfort eating. Prior planning for your trigger moments is vital.

In a nutshell, it involves recognising that you do have control, you just need to take it back. When you stop *reacting*:

Emotion   Automatic behaviour/Eating (hurts you)

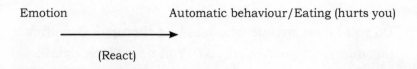

(React)

Give yourself a chance to think, so you can switch off your autopilot and choose what to do:

Emotion   Better Choice (helps you)

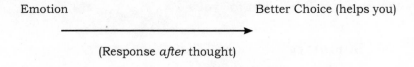

(Response *after* thought)

Part 7 – Keeping It Going
36. 'But My Life Needs To Get A Little Better Before I Can Even Start!'

Firstly, I'd like you to look at this graph. This beautifully demonstrates where you're headed, depending on your daily routine choices. It also shows where you will end up if you keep putting this off.

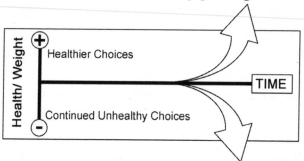

If you're unhappy with your current health and weight right now, accept that it's due to previous choices you've made. These choices have played themselves out over time. This is where you are as a result.

Sometimes, you might have had the best intentions, but made your choices on poor information. Other times, you've made your choices knowing full well they don't help you.

Some choices concerning what action to take can lead to instant, and even dramatic, feedback. For example, if you tell your spouse you're leaving them, the feedback is instant!

However, the feedback from your daily routine choices, about what to eat and what exercise to take, are not instant. The health and weight implications take time to make themselves known.

There are loads of little areas to focus on during your journey to good health. Let's take one example: to continue eating beyond feeling satisfied - or not. This is a relatively easy decision to make, but there's no instant feedback, so perhaps little thought goes into it as a result. It's not like you're not going to put two stone on because of this one occasion of overeating, so there's no big problem here. There's no drama, not like if you told your spouse you were leaving.

Deciding whether or not to eat too much on one occasion is not a dramatic decision. It could be a boring choice, one that nobody else witnesses. It's sometimes difficult to make the right choice when there is no immediate feedback.

The right and wrong choices you make on any given day will have little or no noticeable impact that day, or the day after, or the next one. But it is precisely these small daily decisions, which may seem insignificant, but when compounded over time, will dramatically affect how your health and weight will turn out.

If you overeat most of the 365 days of the year, that adds up to an awful lot over time. Time can be your friend, or your enemy, depending on the small, routine choices you make every day.

Which side of the graph will you be on in a year's time?

Assume you'll be alive and kicking this time next year, regardless of what side of the graph you choose to be on. The big question is: are you going to continue doing the same things you've always done - those things that have got you to where you are now? If so, this means you'll be even unhealthier than you are now. Your health will not stay the same; it will deteriorate over time:

Bad choices + time = deterioration in your health
(+ possible weight gain)

Cast your mind back to part 5, where you learned about metabolism. Your health isn't static. If you don't regularly do things to improve it, it will get worse. There's no escaping this.

By now, you have the tools to be on the other side of the graph. But the potential problem is choice - your choice. It's those small, mundane daily choices within your power that will put you on the other side. It could be the ones that don't seem important at the time, because you tend to look at them in isolation and don't add them all up.

To get onto the other side of the graph, all you have to do is make small but regular and consistent changes. Small and regular changes add up to BIG change when added up and mixed with time. If you dropped only 2lb per month, you would have 24lb less fat this time next year. You'd also have slashed your chances of horrible illness, and I've no doubt you'd feel pretty chuffed with yourself too.

Better choices + time = improvement in your health and weight loss

So, which side of the graph will you be on? It really is down to you. There's a saying you'll be familiar with: *you can lead a horse to water, but you can't make it drink.* I came across an interesting twist on this recently:

You can lead a human to knowledge, but you can't make them think or change.

It's your choice. What's it going to be?

37. What To Do For FAST Results

You've learnt so much already from this book, and you're beginning to accept that this is going to be a process, not a quick fix. That said, if you focus on certain things initially, you'll get quicker results, and I'm pretty sure you want that. I recommend starting with these five areas, but not necessarily starting them all at the same time. If you make this feel like hard work, by attempting to do too much all at once, you'll set yourself up for failure. Be easy on yourself. As long as you're making progressive, small changes, you'll get there (as long as you know where 'there' is).

Number 1 - Where Are You Going?

Imagine you're a pilot and you're in a plane on the runway, ready for take-off. There's a problem, however. You don't know where you're going! Without knowing exactly where you're going there's little point taking off, and if you do, you'll soon be coming back to your starting point.

You HAVE TO decide what you want. This is the bedrock of your journey. You have to give your subconscious something to get hold of, and keep your focus on this. Otherwise your subconscious will work with what it's already programmed with, and where has that got you so far? **Change starts in your mind.** This involves spending some time thinking, there's no way around this bit.

In Part 2 you were introduced to how important your mind-set is, and how to start programming it for success. This part deserves more attention than just one read through. You can't learn how to do everything in it from one quick read. Go through this chapter again, slowly. Spend time thinking about the content and how it relates to what you want for your health and weight. Really nail down your goal and your plan to achieve it. By now, you'll have loads of potential steps you can take, together with everything you've learnt in this book.

Doing this bit starts giving you the confidence that you can really do this, and lose your excess fat. Putting some effort in here will result in you feeling inspired and confident, and this will start carrying you forward towards a slimmer and healthier body.

If you haven't done this bit yet, go back to Part 2 and do it. Get it written out in your notebook, or on your computer, if that works better for you. This is an absolute 'must do' if you want to succeed, and I know you do.

Number 2 – Hydration

Because thirst can be perceived as hunger, if you don't keep yourself well hydrated, you'll end up eating more than you need.

Fat breakdown needs water to be freely available. Your little fat busting enzymes (lipase) need water to break fat down into smaller fatty acids. Make their job easy and straightforward by being well hydrated.

Are you supporting your anabolic metabolism by drinking eight glasses a day? If you aren't doing that yet, ask yourself, why not? What's stopping you doing this? Once you've answered that question, think about how you can overcome that reason and make a change for the better.

Remember, there's no rush. If you don't usually drink any water, you don't need to dive in straight away with the full eight glasses every day. The most important time to hydrate is when you get out of bed, so start there. Gradually build it up.

Number 3 – Seriously Reduce Refined White Carbs

Refined white carbs and sugar cause your body to produce loads of insulin. The more immediate effect of this is fat storage.

Refined white carbs and sugar don't keep you full for long, and they increase your appetite by causing low blood sugar and malnutrition of the smaller nutrients you need.

You will make great progress by cutting down on this rubbish. If you currently eat a lot of this sort of 'food', cut down gradually. Gradually substitute them for healthier options. As you get used to healthier options, slowly add more in and reduce the refined stuff further.

By eating real food you give your body the nutrition it craves. Eat unrefined whole foods that keep you full for a lot longer and which nourish your body. It won't be long before you're feeling more energetic and less hungry.

Number 4 – Eat Right

Your body will let you know when it needs food, but be careful:

- Have you been keeping yourself hydrated? If not, have a drink of water 30 minutes before eating and then gauge your hunger.
- If you're getting hungry quickly after eating, are your current choices driving this – have you been eating nutrient-deficient, refined white carbs?
- If you know you're eating when you're not hungry, why is this? Are you eating because of boredom or emotional reasons? Part 6, which is about comfort and emotional eating, is another area that may need multiple reads and plenty of time spent thinking. Make it a priority to re-read this part if it's relevant to you, and define your plan as to how you're going to start overcoming this.

The hunger scale is so important it's worth repeating:

The Hunger Scale
1 – Feeling faint
2 – Absolutely ravenous
3 – Quite hungry
4 – Peckish
5 – Neutral
6 – Satisfied
7 – Full
8 – Over full
9 – Stuffed and bloated
10 – So full you could vomit
Eat when you notice yourself at 3 or 4

Eat when you notice yourself at 3 or 4. Chew your food well. Enjoy and savour every mouthful. Eating should be pleasure, not a race.

Wherever possible, avoid getting to 1 and 2. When you eat in this state you're highly likely to overshoot the mark and eat too much.

Stop eating before you reach 8 and beyond. Give yourself a chance to do this by eating slowly, and tune into your stomach over what's on your plate. It's really hard to do this if you eat in front of the TV. Your focus is on what you're watching, not what you're doing. If you regularly overeat and get too full, and you eat in front of the TV, turn the TV off while you're eating for at least a month. It's very difficult to learn something new while you're switching your mind off.

If you choose not to switch the TV off while you're eating, ask yourself this: 'Am I choosing TV over my health?' Is watching TV for 15-20 minutes while you eat really that important?

You might be amazed at how much more attention you pay to what's going on inside your mouth, and you'll probably enjoy your food more as a result. You'll be much more likely to notice your 'full' signal before you overeat.

It might help to look at the hunger scale before, and while, you eat. It can take a while to change old habits. In the early days it's helpful to keep reminding yourself, until it sinks in and becomes part of you.

Number 5 – Increasing Your Activity

Where's your fitness at right now? Accept wherever you are with this and jump in at an appropriate level. What I mean by this is, start where you're going to stretch yourself, at least by a little.

If you currently do practically nothing, increase your walking as your first step. Get used to this first. Perhaps get a pedometer to measure how you're doing. Up your game as you get fitter.

If you're already reasonably fit, because you exercise regularly, consider starting the high intensity workouts detailed in part 4. The beauty of this is that you can make great gains with little time input. From there, you can add some strength training, which doesn't take you long either.

Keep a record of your progress in your notebook, because what gets measured is more likely to get done. At some point this will become part of your routine and you'll do it as if on autopilot.

Summary

Concentrating your efforts here is more than enough to really kick start your fat loss at the beginning. As these bits fall into place and gradually become normal for you, you can start slowly incorporating other aspects of the book.

Treat this as a long term project on yourself. If you were embarking on a total renovation of a house, you know it would take more than a week to do, and things have to take place in the right order. The same kind of thing applies here.

38. Keeping Yourself Motivated

Your mind-set is the star player here, because to BE healthy, you have to THINK healthily first:

- You have to become slim and healthy in your mind with your thoughts first.
- To consistently keeping doing what you need to do to be slim and healthy, so that...
- You can **have** a slim and healthy body for the long term.

Your thoughts have to change first. When they do you won't need motivation, you'll be inspired to change and just get on with it like it's the natural thing to do. Yes, it can happen like that when you get your mind-set sorted. That's why this part is so important to your success.

Remember, *you* get more of what your mind is focused on, so by now:

1. You'll have written down your goal in your notebook.

- This is quite specific and conjures up an image and/or feeling in your head when you think about it

2. You'll be reviewing that goal and imagining you've achieved it already. You're doing this regularly because you know this programs your subconscious for success. You will get there with your subconscious on board.

- You imagine what you look like when you've reached your goal
- You imagine what it's like to be in your body, and how good it feels

- You may imagine yourself in some great clothes you'd love to wear
- Pick one thought e.g. a loved one saying how great you look, and use this thought often. Feel it like it's real. The better this thought makes you feel the more effective it will be at programming your subconscious. Spend a minute or two every day on this – just before you get up, or before you go to sleep.
- You don't have to imagine all sorts of different thoughts (but you can do, if you prefer), one particular thought about you when you achieve your goal is enough – repetition is the real key here

3. You're writing your thoughts, your learning, and changes you've made in your notebook. Reviewing this inspires you.

- Flicking through this at times of doubt can really boost your confidence again; that's why it's so important to have this record

Remind yourself how much focus, and how long, it took you to learn to walk, talk, or drive a car? Did you give up when you made a mistake or it felt a bit hard? Or did you keep going and get there at some point? When you treat this stuff in the same way there's no room for failure, only success. Like in other areas of your life, you can do this too.

Learning takes repetition, that's why you can't just read this book once, expect to have the answers and be fixed. Repetition is needed to establish new habits for long term change (otherwise, you'll be at the mercy of your old habits for the rest of your days).

Repetition means reading parts of this book more than once. It involves focusing on the bits that have caught your attention, the bits you've highlighted as you've gone along. It means reviewing your own notes in your notebook.

Are you signed up to my newsletter? By doing so you'll receive regular reminders about information you've learned here, and also new information in my fat loss blogs that will continue to help you. Instead of passively reading these, increase your learning by asking me a question or leaving a comment. I love hearing from readers, and I'm always happy to personally answer questions.

There's everything you need in this book, apart from ongoing support. It would be ideal if you can do this with someone, or even better, a small group of people. Then you could check in with them regularly and support and encourage each other as you go along. People who have support are more likely to do well.

But it can feel lonely if you're the only person you know who's taking your health seriously and making the effort to change. If this is you consider joining my club where you can get access to me every week via my live webinar. (A webinar is like an online seminar or conference that you can watch and listen to on your computer, either live, or on catch up, if you miss it).

These can be your point of contact every week to keep you tuned into your goals and the changes you are making. Being a member of the club also gives you the opportunity to ask me questions. You obviously get the benefit of hearing me answering other people's questions too. This adds massively to your learning and progress.

It takes time to cement the changes needed for long lasting change, and checking in with me every week will help keep your mind on the job. Without this, you may be in danger of falling back into old habits. Staying involved every week will give you a sense of accountability that's invaluable regarding the journey you've begun.

Find out more about the club here
http://uberhealthblog.com/uber-slim-club/

39. Summary

The most important thing, to ensure you stay motivated and see this through, is to NOT overwhelm yourself by doing too much too soon. Focus on the quick hits first:

- Improve your mind-set – this takes regular input from you
- Improve your hydration and quality of carbohydrate intake
- Improve the way you eat (as well as what you eat)
- Gradually incorporate more activity into your day
- Get support – either do this with someone else or consider joining my club where you'll get all the support you need

You've got everything here to achieve the body and health you want; all you have to do is make gradual, small, but consistent changes. You can do this.

Food Ideas
Breakfast Ideas

Smoothie

I use the Kenwood Smoothie 2GO to make my smoothies and I have one most mornings for breakfast. One of the good things about this smoothie maker is that it makes it easy to walk out of the door with your smoothie, if you're not ready to eat first thing, or you haven't got time.

Because of the great quality fat from the avocado and oil it's really filling, and will keep you going for ages. Just put these ingredients into a jug and blend, it only takes a few minutes. Vary fruit. Berries are a great choice because they're lower in sugar than other fruits and packed with essential nutrients.

This is a great way to get a daily dose of raw, nutrient-packed food.

INGREDIENTS

Handful of sprouts
2 handfuls of blueberries
1 banana
1 avocado
1tbsp of Udo's Choice Ultimate Oil Blend
Top up with juice - ideally fresh vegetable or fruit juice, otherwise, shop bought juice

Notes:

- sprouts = sprouted seeds, e.g. lentils or beans (see end of section for more details)
- Udo's Oil = high quality oil that's a great source of essential oils, especially omega 3 (you can get this from www.bodykind.com)

Wheat-free pancake

This is probably more aptly named a fruit omelette.

Mash up one banana to 2 eggs.
Mix the mashed bananas with the eggs.
Melt a small knob of butter in a non-stick pan.
Pour a pancake size amount into the pan.
Cook for a couple of minutes each side until lightly golden.

These are usually sweet enough without anything added.
You can vary the fruit to anything you like.

Other breakfast options

- Poached eggs on spelt or rye toast
- Omelette
- Porridge (perhaps not every day, because it's high carb)

Lunch Ideas

Split pea soup

I often make a big saucepan of this by doubling the quantities. Any not eaten after a few days can be frozen for another occasion.

INGREDIENTS

250gm yellow split peas, soaked for 8 hours
1 onion – chopped
1 medium sweet potato, chopped
3 medium carrots, chopped
750ml of vegetable stock
Salt and pepper to season to taste

METHOD

1. Rinse the split peas and put them into a large saucepan, along with everything else.
2. Bring to the boil then leave to gently simmer until everything is soft, usually about 30 minutes.
3. Blend with a hand blender until smooth

Eat on its own or with spelt or rye bread.

Salad

This is something easy to take to work, or have at home. It makes a nice alternative to sandwiches.

Include any, or all, of these salad ingredients:

A bag of organic salad leaves

Tomatoes

Red pepper

Red onion

Cucumber

Carrots

Radish

Olives

I often do too many steamed veggies the night before, and therefore include these too

Add a salad dressing to make things interesting and tasty (recipe below)

Add your choice of meat, fish, eggs or cheese. Or tinned mackerel is another option.

Other lunch options

- Omelette
- Leftovers from the night before (I often deliberately make too much to make lunch easy the next day)
- A sandwich made with spelt or rye bread

Main Meal Ideas

Chowder

INGREDIENTS

600g/1lb 5oz smoked haddock

1 pint of whole milk

1tbsp of butter

3 sticks of celery, thinly sliced

3 medium leeks, sliced

2 bay leaves

2 medium potatoes - peeled and cut into small cubes

1 pint of fish stock

125g/4oz sweetcorn

150ml single cream or crème fraiche

2tbsp chopped fresh parsley

METHOD

1. Lay the haddock in a deep frying pan and pour over the milk. Cover and bring to the boil. Remove from the heat and leave undisturbed for about 5 minutes, until the haddock is just cooked. Lift the haddock from the milk, remove the skin and bones and flake onto a plate. Keep the milk for later.

2. Heat the butter in a saucepan and add the celery, leeks, potatoes and bay leaves and cook for a couple of minutes. Pour in the stock and the milk. Simmer and cook for about 10 minutes, until the potatoes are soft.

3. Add the haddock, sweetcorn and cream. Season with pepper (it shouldn't need any salt with the fish and stock) and stir in the parsley. Heat through gently and serve.

Chicken with chunky vegetables

Serves 4

INGREDIENTS

250g/9oz shallots
8 small carrots
2 sticks of celery
2 leeks
2tbsp butter
1.5kg/3lb chicken
425ml/3/4pint each of chicken stock and dry white
wine
2 bay leaves
2 sprigs of thyme
Small handful of parsley

METHOD

1. Peel the carrots, and cut in half if large. Trim the
celery and leeks and cut into 5cm lengths.
2. Add the shallot to a frying pan with the butter,
cook over a medium heat until they begin to brown.
Add the rest of the vegetables and cook for another 5
minutes until the vegetables are just golden.
3. Place the chicken in a large pot with a tight fitting
lid and arrange the vegetables around it.
4. Add the chicken stock and the wine.
5. Tuck the bay leaves, thyme and parsley around the
chicken and season with salt and pepper.

6. Cover with the lid and cook on the middle shelf of the oven for an hour and 10 minutes at 170C/Gas 4, or until the juices run clear. Take the lid off for the last 15 minutes.

7. When cooked, take the chicken out and leave to rest for a few minutes. Then carve up and served with steamed vegetables and a small baked potato.

Bouillabaisse (delicious, hearty fish stew)
Serves 4, but easy to double up so that it lasts you a few days

INGREDIENTS

Approx. 450g of mixed white fish, skinned and cubed (e.g. monkfish, haddock, cod, red mullet, etc.)
Approx. 170g of raw, peeled prawns
1 large onion, sliced
1-2 cloves garlic, crushed
4 carrots, thinly sliced
2 bay leaves
Bouquet garni (you can buy these as 'teabags' of herbs, alongside other herbs in your supermarket)
Pinch of saffron (optional)
2 sticks of celery, chopped
2 small leeks, sliced
Fennel bulb, chopped
Bunch of fresh parsley
1/2 pint of fish or vegetable stock
2 tins of chopped tomatoes

1/2 teaspoon cayenne pepper
Unwaxed orange peel
2 tablespoons of Pernod
Few drops of Tabasco sauce

METHOD

1. Gently sauté the onion and garlic in a large, deep pan, until soft. Add the sliced carrots, chopped tomatoes, stock, bay leaves, saffron, and bouquet garni. Bring to the boil and then simmer for about 30 mins with the lid on.
2. Add the leeks and celery and continue to simmer, until the carrots start to go soft. Add salt and pepper to taste.
3. Add the fennel and orange peel and simmer for 10 mins.
4. You may want to set a timer for the next part, so as not to overcook your fish. Firstly, add the firm fish (such as monkfish, swordfish) and cook for 2 mins.
5. Then add the more delicate fish (haddock, cod, mullet) and cook for 5 mins.
6. Add the prawns, cayenne pepper and Pernod (this will give it a lovely aniseed kick) and cook for 2 mins. Stir in the parsley, and you're ready to serve.

Veggie chilli (can be adapted for meat lovers by adding chunks of your preferred meat)

Serves 4, but easy to double up so you have a lovely pot full of healthy food to last a few days.

INGREDIENTS

1 red onion, peeled and cut into big chunks
1/2 red chilli (or more, depending on how hot you like it), deseeded and cut into chunks
1 dried, smoked chipotle chilli (I cheat and put in a teaspoon of Tesco Chipotle Chilli & Smoked Paprika paste, to add a lovely, smoky flavour)
1-2 garlic cloves, crushed
1/2 teaspoon cumin seeds
1 teaspoon smoked paprika
1 + 1/2 tablespoons extra virgin olive oil
Large bunch of fresh coriander - save the stalks
2 peppers, deseeded and chopped
1 large onion, chopped
A big box of mushrooms, halved or quartered
400g tin of chickpeas
400g tin of black beans (or haricot, adzuki, or any types of bean, all easy to find in your local supermarket)
2 tins of chopped tomatoes

METHOD

1. First, make an easy chilli paste in a food processor

or blender. Put the chillies and red onion into your processor, along with the cumin seeds, smoked paprika, extra virgin olive oil (and chilli paste, if you're cheating, like I do). Squash the peeled garlic through a garlic press and add that, along with the stalks from your coriander bunch. Save the leaves for later. Whizz this together in your food processor until it makes a fine paste.

2. Sauté your other onion gently with a bit of butter. When it starts to go soft, add your chilli paste mixture from your food processor. Continue to cook this gently for a few minutes.

3. Add the peppers, mushrooms, and cook for another minute or two. Then add the chopped tomatoes. Give your chick peas and beans a rinse in a colander and add them to the pan. Bring it to a steady boil then turn the heat down. Place the lid on the pan, stirring regularly. Add salt and pepper to taste.

4. Cook in this manner for about 20 mins to half an hour. Just before serving, add the chopped coriander leaves. Serve with brown rice or a large portion of steamed vegetables. Delicious!

Tuna with salsa
Tuna steak served with freshly made salsa, steamed vegetables, and a small portion of boiled potatoes (with butter).

You get most benefit, when it comes to good fats, if you eat fish raw. Sushi isn't my cup of tea, however,

for this reason, I have my steaks on the rare side.
This maximises the benefit but also gives me a meal I
enjoy.

TUNA

Cooking time will vary with the thickness of the steak.
If you're not used to cooking them, it will take a bit
of practice. It's best to risk underdoing it; you can
always cook it a bit more, if necessary. Aim to have a
least a bit of pink in the middle of the steak.

Sprinkle a little sea salt on the steak – both sides.
Also, grind some black pepper over it. Rub in, along
with some butter.

Put into a hot, non-stick frying pan. Each side will
need between 90 seconds and 2 minutes, depending
on the thickness of the steak.

SALSA – mix together all these ingredients and lay
over the cooked tuna:
250gm chopped tomatoes
1 small red onion, finely chopped
1 small red chilli, finely chopped
10cm piece of cucumber, finely chopped
Half a red pepper, finely chopped
2 handfuls of chopped coriander
Juice from half a lime

Other Main Meal Ideas

- Your choice of meat, fish or omelette with a large portion of steamed veg (dark-green leafy ones are best), and small (i.e. 2-3) portion of either boiled new potatoes with butter, or a small jacket potato.

Other Things

Wholegrain spelt loaf

Spelt naturally proves and rises quicker than wheat flour, so bake it as soon as it's doubled in size. If making this in a bread machine use the 'gluten cycle' or 'rapid cycle', but check your machine instructions/ guidelines to be sure.

INGREDIENTS

500gm wholegrain spelt flour
1.5tsp salt
1.5tsp yeast (or 1 sachet)
1tsp sugar
300ml warm water
1tbsp soft butter

METHOD

1. Mix the flour, salt, yeast and sugar together in a large bowl.
2. Add the water and butter and mix into the flour.

Leave the dough for 5 minutes to absorb the water.

3. Knead the dough well until it feels smooth.

4. Leave the dough covered with a clean cloth, in a warm place, until it's doubled in size; it should take about an hour.

5. Turn the dough out onto a floured surface and knead firmly for several minutes

6. Shape the dough and put into a greased (butter) 1kg/2lb bread tin, or shape and place the dough onto a greased baking sheet.

7. Cover again and leave to rise for about 30 minutes in a warm place.

8. Remove the cover and put into a preheated oven for 35-45 minutes at 220C/425F/Gas 7

9. It's ready when the bottom sounds hollow when tapped.

10. Allow it to cool and enjoy with butter.

Healthy salad dressing

This is really healthy. The olive oil is full of good fats that are great for your health. Most bought salad dressings are highly processed and have nothing going for them when it comes to your health.

Using a pestle and mortar, grind together half a clove of garlic, a teaspoon of wholegrain mustard, a pinch of sea salt, and any small amount of any fresh herbs you may have.

Add 6tbsp of extra virgin olive oil and 3tbsp of good quality balsamic vinegar.

Mix together then pour into an empty jam jar. Give it a good shake before use; store in the fridge and it will last you all week.

Guacamole
Serves 4

INGREDIENTS

1 red chilli - optional
1 clove of garlic - optional
A handful of coriander, chopped
2 finely chopped tomatoes
Salt to taste
1 small, finely chopped onion
Juice from half a lime
3 ripe avocados

METHOD

1. In a pestle and mortar, grind the chilli, garlic, coriander, salt and onion into a fine paste. Add the lime juice.
2. Mash the avocados. Add in the paste you've made, and the chopped tomatoes.

This can be used as a dip, a side dish, or spread on

such as Ryvitas as a snack.

How to sprout

This is really easy to do and gives you something super healthy to add to smoothies and salads.

You'll need a sprouting tray. These are small, and will easily tuck out of the way on your kitchen surface. Get a cheap and easy one; I found this one on Amazon, it should be fine to get you started if you want to try this: A.Vogel BioSnacky Large Germinator by A Vogel.

Take your chosen seed and soak overnight. Rinse and place into the tray. Rinse the seeds twice per day. In a few days they'll start to sprout; at this stage, they're ready to eat.

There are lots of things you can sprout, including:
• Mung beans
• Green lentils
• Brown lentils
• Chickpeas

Buy packets of dried lentils or beans from the supermarket. Put a handful in a smoothie or over the top of a salad.

These are just a few ideas as to healthy things to eat. This is an area I'll expand on during my weekly webinars. Within these webinars, you can also share recipe ideas you've had, or check with me as to how healthy a particular meal is.

A common theme running through these recipes and suggestions is real food. You can easily build on this by sticking to this principle.

Glossary

Adrenal glands – you have two and they sit on top of each of your kidneys. They produce a variety of hormones, in particular those that cause stress in your body

Amino acids – the small building blocks of protein
Antioxidant – a substance that protects cells in your body from damage by free radicals

BMI (Body Mass Index) – a simple calculation that's commonly used to indicate whether you are a healthy weight for your height. In my opinion, it's not very helpful

Cirrhosis of the liver – permanent loss of healthy liver cells from scarring, due to damage

Degenerative disease - the function or structure of affected tissues or organs increasingly deteriorate over time, whether due to normal bodily wear or lifestyle choices, such as a lack of exercise or poor eating habits

Diabetes – a condition where you don't produce enough insulin, and therefore cannot control your blood sugar levels

Diuretic – a substance that promotes the production of urine

Endothelial cells – the cells that line the surface of structures like the lungs and digestive track

Enzyme – a biological catalyst that brings specific biochemical changes

Fatty acids - the small building blocks of fats and oils

Free radicals – substances that combine with healthy cells and tissues, damaging them in the process

Glucose – a simple sugar that's an important energy source in your body; mainly comes from carbohydrates

Gluten – a protein found in wheat, barley, rye and other grains

Glycogen – glycogen is stored glucose; it's found in your muscles and liver

Hormone – substances often made out of protein that act as messengers within your body

IBS (Irritable Bowel Syndrome) – the diagnosis given to people when no other cause can be found for symptoms including abdominal pain, constipation, diarrhoea, bloating

Insulin – a hormone produced by your pancreas that keeps your blood glucose within safe levels

Leptin – a hormone released by fatty tissues

Neurotransmitter – a brain messenger that communicates messages within the brain

Oestrogen – a hormone responsible for female characteristics

Pancreas – a gland that sits behind your stomach. It's vital in the digestive process, producing many digestive juices and enzymes. It also produces insulin.

Serotonin – a neurotransmitter involved in the controlling of our moods and sleep

Testosterone – a hormone responsible for male characteristics

About The Author, Dr Julie, And Her Uber Slim Programme

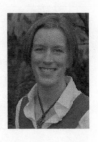

I'm Julie Coffey and I would like to thank you for reading this book.

I am a doctor working within the NHS in the UK. I'm a General Practitioner and I qualified as a doctor in 1994, and have been working as a GP since 1998. I work mainly in Sheffield.

From an early age, I wanted to do something worthwhile. I trained as a doctor because I wanted to learn, and I wanted to help people.

I've always been interested in health but I began to find the medical community's approach to health and wellbeing increasingly frustrating. The predominant focus on treating and managing illness was to supply pills, with little emphasis on maintaining or regaining natural vitality.

When it comes to weight loss, the limit of many doctors' advice to patients was to eat less and do more. This, coupled with the pressure of body image through the media, led me to see many people continuing to destroy their health from years of following bad advice, or by continuing with diets.

In my mid to late thirties I started to develop osteoarthritis in my knees. I knew that conventional medicine had little to offer me.

I was worried about this as I'm an active person, and even things like walking became quite uncomfortable at times. I wondered if I'd get to a point where I wouldn't be able to do the things I loved - like skiing.

I decided to stop worrying, and instead, put all my energy into discovering a solution. I wasn't going give up my ability to enjoy life without a fight.

I started reading endless books and research papers, and felt like I was starting my health education again, almost from scratch. There was so much I didn't know. I found this new knowledge exciting and fascinating.

With my medical background, I began to design a regime for my body based on the learning I'd undertaken. I immersed myself in developing a natural health programme that helped me make diet and lifestyle changes. My knees began to get better and were far more comfortable. I also lost the stubborn pounds that had been creeping up on me over a few years.

My medical background allowed me to sort fact from fiction and create a change in my own lifestyle. The effects were so dramatic, and created such freedom for me, that I was inspired to create my unique online weight-loss course, 'Uber Slim', so that others could benefit from the hard work I'd done to find the answers.

So How Does My Uber Slim Programme Work?

Uber Slim is all about getting back to, and maintaining, your natural state of health – which is good health.

Uber Slim builds on the information I've shared in this book. It gives you all the facts and structure you will need to rapidly change the way you look and feel forever, in a bite-sized way.

And on top of that, Uber Slim gives you direct access to me. This means you have your own personal coach to answer questions and help you through the tough times.

You won't find any advice here that I'm not doing myself already. And, as a doctor, I never do anything without knowing that it's the right thing for my health.

The benefit of being a doctor is that I know a lot about how the body works; I know what's happening when it goes wrong. I know what pharmaceutical drugs do.

I'm also familiar with reading scientific literature and studies and interpreting them.

I only take on board lifestyle and diet changes if I'm convinced they're the right thing to do and I will get the benefits.

Through my unique Uber Slim programme, you can benefit from everything I've learned, safe in the knowledge that it's coming from a highly qualified, practising health professional.

To get the benefits of Uber Slim right now, and to continue your journey, visit http://uberhealthblog. com/uber-slim-program/

Find out more about the weekly motivation club here http://uberhealthblog.com/uber-slim-club/

You can also use the contact page to drop me an email with any questions you may have before getting involved.

It's going to be a great journey, but you have to act now, before you talk yourself out of making a positive change to your life.